Visualise the New You

FIRST EDITION

Wayne Lambert

VISUALISE THE NEW YOU

By Wayne Lambert

Certified Personal Trainer

Certified Nutrition Specialist

Certified Life Coach

C.E.O & Founder – Whole Body Workshop

Author of Psychology of weight loss and Exercise your whole body at home

Disclaimer: The information provided by this book is not a substitute for a face-to-face consultation with your physician and should not be construed as individual medical advice. If a condition persists, please contact your physician. The testimonials on the website are individual cases and do not guarantee that you will get the same results. The content is provided for personal and informational purposes only. This book is not to be construed as any attempt to either prescribe or practice medicine. Neither is the book to be understood as putting forth any cure for any type of acute or chronic health problem. You should always consult with a competent, fully licensed medical professional when making any decision regarding your health. The owners of this company will use reasonable efforts to include up-to-date and accurate information, but make no representations, warranties, or assurances as to the accuracy, currency, or completeness of the information provided. The owners of this company shall not be liable for any damages or injuries resulting from your reliance upon any information provided in this book. All rights reserved. No part of this publication may be reproduced, transmitted, transcribed, stored in a retrieval system or translated into any language, in any form, by any means, without the written permission of the author.

ISBN 9780 9 5614 940 4

Important
The author assumes no responsibility for any consequence relating directly or indirectly to any action or inaction you take based on the information,
services or other material contained or implied in this book.
There are no implied endorsements of any product mentioned herein.

I dedicate this book to my late grandfather
Lesley James Lambert

Who was and still is an inspiration to me. I know he is happy now that he is reunited with his wife, my wonderful late Grandmother May Lambert whom we also miss so very much.

This book is also dedicated to your
Permanent weight loss success,

May Visualise the New You provide you with
everything you desire.

ACKNOWLEDGEMENTS

As with every person who finds the time to write a book I am no different with regards to how many people I have to thank for their individual assistance in making it happen. I am extremely grateful to my current employers who allowed me to take medical leave on completion of my knee operation and Alan Caine my previous manager who was supportive throughout. Having had that 3 months rest period gave me enough time to put together this book amongst starting my own business and building my own website www.wholebodyworkshop.com.

I thank my friends, relatives and close family, starting of course with my father Terry, my brother Darren and sister-in-law Barbie who have all been there for me when I needed them most. I need to thank Laila who has more than changed my life over the last 6 months in more ways than one and I thank her for her unconditional support in everything I do.

Support in the early stages especially, goes to my cousin Melanie who let me know 'how it is' regarding what goes on in the mind of someone who wants to lose weight. I would also like to thank Paul Day, a close friend and ex Royal Marine who speaks so very highly of me in his foreword within this book and yet he himself has done so many great things since leaving the military, not to mention graduating with honours from one of the top universities in the world, where he studied physiotherapy. Personally I have learned so much from him, especially related to his consistent professionalism and support for others.

A special thankyou must go to Sally Balsdon who is featured in all of the photos; Sally gave up her spare time to assist me in the early stages when I was writing the content for the exercise chapters. Even though there was a shortage of volunteers there were also not many people who would have met the grade and so on that note I couldn't have wished for anyone better to stand pride of place within my very first book, so I thank her for that.

Apologies to anyone I may have forgotten to mention.

TABLE OF CONTENTS

FOREWARD

I have known Wayne since our days in the Armed Forces together, and throughout this time he has been one of the most determined and dedicated people I have had the pleasure to know. He practices all that he preaches and also has the integrity to admit if he has not done so for any given reason. As a friend and a previous work colleague Wayne is and was always 100% supportive and reliable. He is also the most talented lateral thinker I have known, thus making any problem his family or friends may encounter easily resolved, a true friend in every sense of the word.

This book is part of 'Whole Body Workshop' a company Wayne has put together to address the whole person in their journey towards whatever goal they wish to achieve. Indeed weight loss may be the primary goal most individuals who read this text wish to achieve, however his book, a tool within the company, will be able to assist you in all your life goals as it addresses the psychological aspects as well as the physiological, in consequence empowering the reader to transfer these principles to other aspects of their life. As already mentioned this book is a guide to empower yourself to become the individual you would like to be, educating every reader allowing them to make the correct choices for themselves. Throughout this book, at the beginning of each subject, Wayne provides you with the real facts of the advantages and disadvantages of the given subject. Most of this is also backed by current literature and statistics, which allows you to research and analyse further, encouraging you to become more educated in the given subject, therefore providing you with the ability to make your own judgements.

Wayne starts from the very beginning, which is how to prepare psychologically; he provides many strategies on how to prepare you psychologically, thus being a strategy for everybody out there. Wayne also provides the reader with tasks, which allows the reader to become an integral player in the transition they require from the very beginning. Wayne discusses the nutritional subjects in a no punches pulled manor, quickly pointing out the health risks of a poor diet and quashing many myths about food that are beneficial to us all. But he doesn't just give statements; he educates the reader, again allowing the reader to make their own decisions. Throughout the movement and exercise components of this book you can really sense Wayne's enthusiasm for this subject. Again he tells you how it is, he looks at the reasons why many people don't exercise, then gives the benefits on why you should, which quickly make those reasons why many people don't exercise appear insignificant excuses. The difference between exercise and diet alone and the benefits of bringing them together are outlined, which assists in bringing some of the messages of this book together. Wayne will agree that there is much more to each subject than in this book, but Wayne has given enough information to empower each individual on the path to lose body fat and become much healthier, in a nice, to the point manner that each and every one of us can relate to. As we progress through our training regimes of fitness and attaining goals, it's not unusual to experience small setbacks at any time, albeit from lack of motivation or by injury.

Many people when injured become extremely frustrated as injury generally occurs when their training is going very well. However to recover from injury, a time of rehabilitation is required. Although at times rehabilitation can be frustrating as this will be governed by the type of injury and the timings of tissue healing. However rehabilitation can open up ideas and regimes not thought of previously that can be incorporated in to an individual's normal training increasing their programme.

Rehabilitation can require lots of psychological strength and patience, this text will provide the reasons behind rehabilitative requirements, and this will allow the reader to reason and motivate themselves which can be frustrating times. Conversely when the injury has resolved, you will feel a sense of achievement by having the autonomy to rehabilitate yourself, which in turn will increase your, self efficacy, promoting more confidence to approach life's goals.

I hope everyone who reads this book finds what they are seeking, and experience, like those of us who have the pleasure of knowing him, what it is like to be introduced to Wayne's way of thinking.

- Paul Day
BSC (Hons) MCSP, SRP, Dip FTST

Who I am and what I can teach you

Since a very young age I have been extremely physically active what with taking up boxing, joining the British Royal Marines at a very young age and entering many fitness competitions throughout the years. Fitness competitions still continue to give me a purpose to keep fit and provide me with drive and ambition. When I start a project I give 110% of my time and effort which is something that I believe is the only way to be successful in all that you do. Success has come my way via winning all of my boxing fights and becoming a boxing coach alongside Paul Denholm (founder of OMG fitness and author of boxing secrets revealed which is based around his website www.boxingsecretsrevealed.com) together we coached a large military boxing team and managed to win the whole competition quite easily.

Whilst serving in the military for 13 years I travelled the world on various operations and many years later managed to specialise as a physical training instructor. Further study also gave me the opportunity to become a rehabilitation therapist working alongside physiotherapists. My continued interest within the health and fitness industry led me to gain many qualifications before leaving the Royal Marines to which helped me gain a worthy position as fitness director of a company within the United States of America. After my mission was completed in America I moved to Dubai to work as a physical training advisor for the military which again was an enormous challenge but a great achievement. In between jobs I have assisted 1000's of clients achieve their goals whether it be weight loss, optimum performance in sport, strength gains or just simple lifestyle changes. My sole aim since leaving school was to give my knowledge to others and that was my inspiration to write my book visualise the new you and to create a company where I could provide a weight consultancy and performance coaching service based around my website www.wholebodyworkshop.com. Every single day I assist people in achieving their goals whether it be via life coaching, personal training or otherwise.

My main objective in life has been to help others and therefore my aim is always to continuously gain qualifications within the health and fitness industry. I truly believe that if a person wants to achieve great things in their chosen industry then their continued education should never end. Clearly we will never know everything in this life but we can still endeavour to know just a little bit of everything in order to stay current and of course to share information with anyone who needs it.

Why I know this book will help you achieve success

So, how can this book help you achieve everything you desire? Well, there is always a punch line and my punch line is this:

In September of 2001, I left the British military and with that transformation and many others, I became less active and I actually picked up a few injuries from thinking that I could do the same sports that I did when I was a teenager when I was actually in my early to mid-thirties. I couldn't train as hard, especially any cardiovascular work and, through time, I actually had to undergo surgery on my knee. All of these factors had an effect on my weight. I was eating the same as I always had and I quite simply assumed that I could do everything that I did as a boy when, in reality, I was in my mid-thirties and inactive. The weight kept creeping on until one day a friend told me how my body had changed and by then it seemed a little too late, especially as I hadn't even noticed my weight creeping up myself. So there you have it. My first negative thought in so many years. I was sure it was too late. Weeks later I decided immediate action was required, but suddenly all of my personal training and nutrition qualifications didn't seem to make it any easier to get started and to proceed to where I wanted to get to. Actually, if you speak to people in the health and fitness industry (the honest ones) you will find that 90% of them don't practice what they preach. To summarise, as a child I was led down the path of joining the military due to my grandfather being in the Army, he taught me many things, especially to think that anything I desired in this life was possible. So I went forward with my life and began visualising about what I wanted, positively thinking about what I desired and started setting my very own personal goals to get where I wanted. Regarding the weight loss, I knew that I had to work around my injury and through my grandfathers imbedded thought processes I knew psychologically that I could lose the weight. After a short while I lost the majority of the weight that I set out to lose and I remained at the maintenance phase thereafter, at least until my knee was better and I could progress accordingly. Unfortunately, the majority of people that are over their natural weight are waiting for that miracle pill, a new diet that actually works, or they believe that a cream or massage belt will get rid of cellulite or tone the body. This book will change that mindset and create a path for new thoughts, new habits and, ultimately, a new you. The Lifestyle Challenges included within this book are not rocket science, they are quick, easy-to-follow tasks that will help you, guide you, and lead you to wherever it is you want to go. There is no limit as to how far you can go, so long as you are safe. You can stop the plan and continue to maintain it wherever you choose. The plan can be kick started after a short break for e.g. summer holidays or Christmas time, as long as you maintain what you had before you stopped. You can pick up where you left off and even change it a little if you are feeling that you've reached a plateau or you are a little bored. The plan is flexible but with guidelines. Stick to the basics and the rest will follow very easily with little effort…just focus!

This book is structured in such a way that it guides you in the right direction from the very beginning and ensures that you are not alone throughout the process of getting to where you need to get to in all that you desire. I can safely say that I couldn't have achieved any of those things without a strategy. That strategy was belief, belief through positive thinking, visualisation and setting personal goals.

- You will…have your own strategy;
- You will…maintain your own belief;
- You will…be more positive;
- You will…visualise what you want and
- You will…have your very own goals to get to where you want to get to.

This book will guide you all the way.

HOW I CAN SET YOU ON THE RIGHT TRACK

"A march of a thousand kilometres begins with a single step."

- Chairman Mao

Things you should know first – Benefits & risks

Risks -
It will be no surprise to you that the percentage of the world in need of weight loss is extremely high, not to mention the amount of money spent on weight loss products per year is astronomically high as well. In fact, the cost is in the billions and getting higher. Once considered a problem only in high-income countries, being overweight and obese is now dramatically on the rise in low and middle income countries, particularly in urban settings. The latest World health organisation projections indicate that at least one in three of the world's adult population is overweight and almost one in ten is obese. Overweight means that they are above their natural weight and obese meaning that they are over fat.

The (W.H.O) world health organisation's latest projections indicate that, globally in 2005:

- Approximately 1.6 billion adults (age 15+) were overweight;

- At least 400 million adults were obese and

- At least 20 million children under the age of 5 years were overweight.

W.H.O further projects that by 2015, approximately 2.3 billion adults will be overweight and more than 700 million will be obese.

FACT
Billions of people each year go on some form of diet that, quite frankly, puts the body into starvation mode, resulting in certain effects on the body, including:

- Fewer fat releasing and fat burning enzymes being released;

- Fewer hormones that tell your brain you are full are released;

- Hormones for fat burning crash;

- Muscle is cannibalised by your own body and

- Hormones controlling appetite cause ravenous cravings.

Body mass index (BMI) & health risk –
The BMI predicts body fat and disease risk better than the popular height-weight tables. A high BMI links to increased risk of death from all causes.

Certain people should not use BMI to infer being overweight or relative disease risk. These people are competitive athletes, body builders, pregnant or lactating women, growing children or sedentary elderly adults.

Body mass index (BMI) represents the ratio of body mass (weight) to stature (height) squared.

BMI = Body mass divided by stature – squared (a calculator will be placed on the website for you)

In June of 1998 the first federal guidelines were released for identifying, evaluating and treating overweight and obesity.

The classifications on BMI are as follows:

Classification	BMI Score	Health risk
Underweight	18.5	
Normal	18.5-24.9	
Overweight	25.0-29.9	Minimal 25.0 / Low 25-27 / Moderate 27-30
Obesity class I	30.0-34.9	High 30-<35
Obesity class II	35.0-39.9	Very high 35-<40
Extreme obesity	>40.0	>40 Extremely high

Benefits –
The benefits of you losing weight personally will be very similar to the next person's benefits. For example, you'll both be looking good, feeling good, be able to do more things physically and have an improved quality of life, including raised self esteem and less depression. But just look at all the health benefits there are from you losing weight. You reduce your risk of heart disease; your cholesterol comes down, particularly the bad type (LDL), while the heart protective good cholesterol (HDL) goes up significantly. Weight loss can reduce the risk of osteoarthritis, gout and even some cancers, including endometrial, breast and colon, to name but a few. All of these conditions can cause premature death and substantial disability.

In addition to all of these benefits, blood pressure and sugar levels come down, which is particularly helpful for diabetics. Plus, there are all the side benefits, such as less tiredness, back pain, joint pain, sweating, breathlessness, snoring, infertility, menstrual irregularities, urinary leakage, etc.

The only sure, safe way to lose your excess weight and keep it off is Mother Nature's way. Your body has built-in, natural fat-burners but, through bad nutrition, these fat-burners become dysfunctional, dormant or plain lazy. That's why you're overweight and the only way you can lose weight and keep it off is to get your natural fat-burners functioning normally and at peak efficiency again. This book will show you how.

You no longer have to listen to gimmicks & lies

The reason why so many millions of people choose to spend their hard earned money on weight loss products and gimmicks is very simple - because of advertising. They all offer a quick fix solution to people's problems and even claim that whatever the product is, it has been scientifically proven to work. Don't you think that if it was genuine, whoever discovered it would be very close to being the world's richest person alive? I must confess, though, that the adverts and promotional stunts do actually sound appealing and I can understand why people choose that route through belief and trust. The fact is that according to the international journal of obesity, weight loss is currently a $150 billion dollar industry, and that's just in the United States and Europe alone. Can you imagine what the figure is on a global front? So do millions of people who believe that somehow, as if by waving a magic wand, they will be thin and firm?

Unwilling or unable to lose weight through diet and exercise, people turn to weight-loss gimmicks ranging from pills that supposedly let them eat unlimited pasta to wearing rubber suits that make them sweat while they sleep.
According to Judith Willis, editor of the United States Food and Drug Administration (FDA) Drug Bulletin, "The most current diet gimmicks of today seem to fall into two categories and they are: (1) Custom garments or body wraps that claim to "melt" fat away in a short time, and (2) Pills that supposedly curb appetites without side effects, or allow dieters to eat normally or more than normal and still lose weight. The pills are usually touted as the product of some previously undiscovered process."

Who can blame these people for being lured by the promise of losing unwanted pounds without doing anything more strenuous than popping a pill or wrapping up the offending flesh? Who can resist advertisements for body wraps that promise "to burn away fat even while you sleep," to "lose 4-6 inches the first day?"

Most medical experts agree that such treatment will cause a loss of inches and perhaps pounds due to profuse perspiration. But the reductions are temporary and the fluid is soon replaced by drinking or eating. But rapid and excessive fluid loss is potentially dangerous because it can bring on severe dehydration and can upset the (homeostasis) balance of important electrolytes in the body.

Through gimmicks and lies, the consumer is being tricked into spending their hard earned money on things that, quite simply, don't work. Fortunately for you there is only one way to lose weight and successfully keep it off. You are about to discover the secret that others before you have already encountered.

Find out why people fail & know the risks

Conventional diets just don't work. Approximately five out of six people who try to lose weight fail and a very high percentage of those who do succeed in losing weight gain all the weight back within two years. If you drop your calories and go hungry, forcing your body to lose weight, your body will fight back. This is your bodies built in "intelligence." It reacts as if you are starving your body and will do everything it can to preserve your fat. When you lose weight by starving yourself, you lose important muscle, bone, fluids, and even vital organ mass. What is not widely known is that the risk of health problems starts when someone is only very slightly overweight and that the likelihood of problems increases as someone becomes more and more overweight. Many of these conditions cause long-term suffering for individuals and families. In addition, the costs for the health care system can be extremely high. What people need to ask themselves is "how long did it take me to put this weight on?" And the answer is more than likely going to be "over a long period of time." The difference being that most people don't even notice the weight "creeping" up before it's actually too late and when it comes to losing it, they all of a sudden expect to actually see it disappearing before their very eyes and because they don't, they give up because it's taking too long.

Whatever attempts people have tried in the past to lose weight, they have either been lied to or they have demanded too much weight loss too soon and, therefore, the expectations have been set far too high. The time that it took to put on weight would ultimately have depended on how active that person was during that period of weight gain and the probability would be that they were quite active at a younger age, therefore it would have taken a long time to put it on and, unfortunately, they are now more than likely living an inactive lifestyle. In short, your body is too smart for short-term quick fixes to ever work because your body will always fight back to maintain a natural balance or, as it is called, "homeostasis."

For every crash diet you go on or diet pill you take, there will always be an equal or greater valley or low point, which basically means that if you over-stimulate, your body can respond by slowing down your natural metabolic rate (i.e. your body's fat burners) to compensate. As a result, when you stop the diet or using the stimulant, your metabolism is slower than ever and you gain back any weight you lost and more.

Those people with what we call "quick fix disease" want to take a pill, go to sleep and wake up skinny. These people are forever on a quest to bypass hard work and find short cuts to health and fitness goals that normally take months or years to attain.

Discover realisation

Generally, health and fitness seekers think they can get twice the results in half the time. Some of the things they want are:

- Weight loss without dieting;

- Fitness without exercise and

- Perfect health while eating, drinking and smoking. whatever they want.

These above beliefs are quite simply unrealistic and will only set you up for failure. Weight loss is easy but needs a little of your effort. Perhaps the biggest realisation of all, for most people, is that all the excuses in the world won't get them to lose weight.

Below are some of the most common excuses:

a. I have big bones;

b. I have a slow metabolism;

c. I have a glandular problem;

d. My hormones are imbalanced;

e. I have a thyroid disorder;

f. My being obese is through genetic influences and

g. 'I hardly eat a thing' syndrome.

Often, the only difference between success and failure with weight loss is how much you want to succeed but, if you are motivated enough, you will have the strength to deal with any circumstances without excuses. You will find ways to deal with whatever life throws at you and, although you might slip up now and again, it hopefully won't be a regular occurrence. One way of increasing your motivation is to have strong enough reasons to succeed and make a note of the reasons why you want to lose weight. If you can find about ten good reasons why you hate being fat or reasons why you no longer want to be overweight, then you can focus on why you want to reach your target and visualise how good life will be when you have achieved your desires. Think about how you will look when that moment arises and of course, how you will feel.

What you need to understand is that, for the majority of overweight people, if you consume more calories than you burn then your weight increases. Yet if you burn more calories than you consume, guess what? It really is that simple!

Prepare yourself

Preparing to lose weight can be the most important part of the whole process. It not only lines you up for success but it also lets all those around you know that you mean business.

So, what can you do to prepare yourself?

- Replace your kitchen with only foods that nourish your body without adding extra pounds, like fresh vegetables and high-calcium foods, such as genuinely low-fat yoghurt, genuinely low-fat cheese and omega-3 eggs;

- Purchase a case of mineral water and fresh limes or lemons to ensure hydration;

- Get rid of foods with extra calories, such as snacks like crisps, cookies and processed foods and

- Purchase some adequate sportswear, an exercise mat and maybe a set of different size rubber weights. Even a personal stereo to take you away from it all, anything that will make your start a permanent one.

Fussy eaters

If you are a fussy eater then you can get your intake of fruit and vegetables through a pill. There is, of course, no substitute for a good diet but there are new supplements on the market that come close. (1) Flavonoid complex. (2) Cruciferous-plus. (3) Mixed carotenoid complex, which is not to be taken by smokers (Packer and Colman, 1999). Until you cover all angles and fully prepare, there is no point beginning because you will surely find some excuse not to continue. Perhaps you should even buy the dress or suit that you want to fit into when you have achieved your goal; it all helps with the process.

Lasting weight loss, however, isn't just about the body because your mind must be on-board too and throughout the whole process from beginning to end, you have to be honest with yourself. If you want to start with good intentions, you should write a journal about your wishes and desires for where you will be in three months, six months and a year. This book will certainly help you do just that, step-by-step.

According to recent breakthroughs in neuroscience, goal setting, visualisation, positive thinking and the law of attraction are all methods that work. Scientists who have worked with the visual parts of the brain have identified ways to filter out all those things that are unimportant and to call our conscious attention to things that are important involved with reaching our goals.

Imagine the brain is like a computer, waiting for a program to be installed, with the subconscious mind ready to carry out any instructions you give it. Over the years, many of us have picked up negative thoughts with programmed beliefs, habits and automatic behaviour. You may or may not know this but the brain cannot differentiate between real practices and practices that are vividly imagined. Thinking positive and starting with small changes will ensure that your changes become long-term but they should be based on loving yourself and not depriving your body. Even attempting to replace certain late night food choices with an exercise class will help you.

Remember though, if this is what you will change, it's important for you to think about how, when, where and with whom you will begin this new exercise class. Whichever way you choose to change, setting a start date is the first phase of putting your plan in motion because having a start date signals the beginning of the new you.

Putting it on your calendar, on your mirror, on the fridge or on your PDA will all help you and not let you forget what it is you are trying to accomplish. Think of it as your most important appointment. But remember, this is an appointment for your health and for your new life.

How you should distribute your time

Before you shift your habits, it's a good idea to determine where your energy goes. You should draw your own pie chart that shows how you spend your time. How much of the pie goes to work, your computer, your family, your friends and not forgetting the all important YOU time? How might you reallocate your energy to make room for change?

A PIE CHART JUST FOR YOU

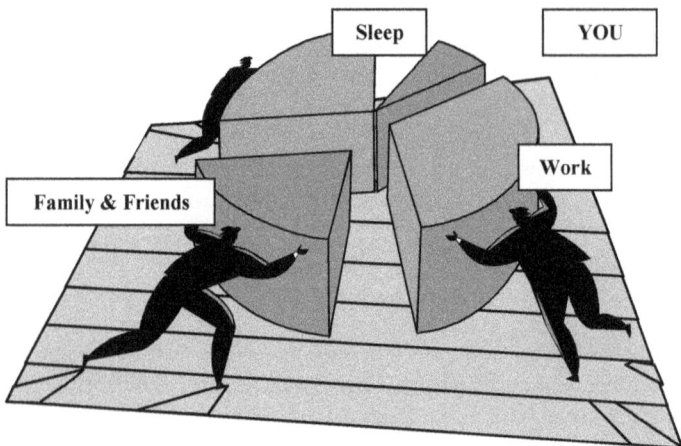

Make a little more time for yourself as and when you can. If it helps, let people around you know what help you need from them and how this will affect you when you are successful.

- The majority of people work an average of 8 hrs;

- We need to sleep for a minimum of 6-8 hours;

- Family and friends depend on your attention and

- Time for yourself is small, but you must have it.

Time should never be the issue for not being able to achieve what you want in your life. Remember, there are 24 hours in each day and that accounts for 1,440 minutes, so you can definitely slot yourself in there somewhere.

In the next chapter, we will show you how to change your thoughts, overwrite old negative programming and only then can we install a positive new program into your subconscious.

SMART STRATEGIES REVEALED TO GET YOU STARTED

"A good way to change somebody's attitude is to change your own."

- George Burns

Dispel the myths

Before we begin with this easy-to-follow system, we have to demolish, destroy and quite literally get rid of all past thoughts about weight loss. Of course I'm referring to all the myths, lies, unrealistic expectations and promises that you have been told or have even heard about through others. Once these are gone from your mind and the record has been set right, only then can you proceed further and replace those thoughts with the honest truth alongside realistic strategies for your successful, long-term weight loss journey.

A few myths revealed:

- Fad diets work for permanent weight loss;

- Skipping meals is a good way to lose weight;

- "I can lose weight while eating anything I want"

- Eating after 8 p.m. causes weight gain;

- Natural or herbal weight-loss products are safe and effective;

- Nuts are fattening and you shouldn't eat them if you want to lose weight;

- Eating red meat is bad for your health and will make it harder to lose weight;

- Starches are fattening and should be limited when trying to lose weight and

- Low-fat or no fat means no calories.

There are many more myths out there but the most common ones were selected for you.

Once you have all Your Own personal myths out of your head you can proceed to the first stage of the Lifestyle Challenges, which involves releasing from within your own personal reasons for wanting to lose weight.

Release your reasons from within

Lifestyle Challenge 1

Make a note of the reasons why you want to lose weight. Find about ten good reasons why you no longer want to be overweight. Then you can focus on why you want to reach your target and visualise how good life will be when you have achieved your desires, how you will look when that moment arises and, of course, how you will feel.

1.   I want to lose weight.....................................

2.   I want to lose weight.....................................

3.   I want to lose weight.....................................

4.   I want to lose weight.....................................

5.   I want to lose weight.....................................

6.   I want to lose weight.....................................

7.   I want to lose weight.....................................

8.   I want to lose weight.....................................

9.   I want to lose weight.....................................

10.   I want to lose weight.....................................

Use words like "because I want," "in order to" and "so I can," but do not continue until you have written down your reasons, or cut them out to keep safe. Trust me when I say that you are already on your way to success, you just have to have faith.

Example: "I want to lose weight so I can walk on the beach and feel comfortable without people staring at me."

Embrace positive thinking

If you have attempted weight loss before, only for the same body fat to return or if you have had the same health problems with the same negative results, then you may have been unconsciously running old negative programs in your head and re-enforcing them with negative thought patterns.

Some examples of negative thoughts are:

•   I will never be able to lose this weight;

•   I won't be able to get into this exercise routine;

- I can't control my eating and

- It must be in my genes, so I give up.

Before you begin you have to demolish, destroy and quite literally get rid of all past negative thoughts about weight loss, including everything you have told yourself in your head or have heard from others.

Once these have gone from your mind and the record has been set straight, only then can you proceed further to replace those negative thoughts with positive ones and a realistic strategy for your successful, long-term weight loss journey.

Lifestyle Challenge 2
In order to successfully change your attitude towards food and drink you must write down a minimum of ten of your own phrases, phrases that you will need to repeat as often as you can throughout the day and throughout the initial twenty one days (non-stop).

The results will be powerful, you'll see.
Some examples of positive self talk phrases are:

- I promise myself not to eat fatty or sweet foods when I am tired or stressed;

- I will have more energy when I cut my fat and sugar intake and increase exercise;

- I will eat more high fibre and low fat foods that I like;

- I can eat often and still lose weight;

- I can handle stress without eating food, especially things I shouldn't be eating;

- I am willing to try a healthy eating and exercise plan to lose and keep off excess fat;

- I know how important water is, so I will drink more of it and

- I will become leaner, healthier and happier after today.

The prevalence of obesity has been on the increase and on the whole, improvements in patient education have not led to the desired outcome of weight maintenance, let alone weight loss.

In more recent decades, behaviour modification approaches have also incorporated strategies from cognitive therapy, which have involved the identification and modification of 'dysfunctional' thinking patterns and consequent negative mood states, hence the term "cognitive behaviour therapy" (CBT).

There is increasing interest in adopting CBT approaches to achieve more modest and sustainable weight loss and improved psychological well being (Liao KL, 2000.)

Your very own positive self talk phrases:

1.	I..

2.	I..

3.	I..

4.	I..

5.	I..

6.	I..

7.	I..

8.	I..

9.	I..

10.	I..

Use powerful words, such as "I can," "I will," and "I am," unless of course the sentence dictates otherwise. These phrases should go with you everywhere and try to place them wherever you can see them. These should be written down now or once you have read the relevant chapters, which will help you.

Example: "I will lose weight because I am more motivated now than ever before and I will not give up until I have."

Visualise how you want to be

When you hold and concentrate on a picture in your mind of how you would like something to be, it ultimately becomes your reality. To visualise losing weight you need to hold a picture in your mind of your ideal body, whether it is by using an old photograph or a magazine picture to help you visualise. The clearer your picture is, the more successful you will be and only then can you spend some time each day thinking of yourself as already having and owning what your image is portraying - this new, improved you. Over time, this will bring you closer to your weight loss goals by working on your subconscious mind to achieve the desired results. Suddenly fast food, sweets, cans of coke and all those desserts will seem less tempting and long walks will seem more fun, but only because of what is in line with the 'set point' you are visualising.

Basics of Visualisation

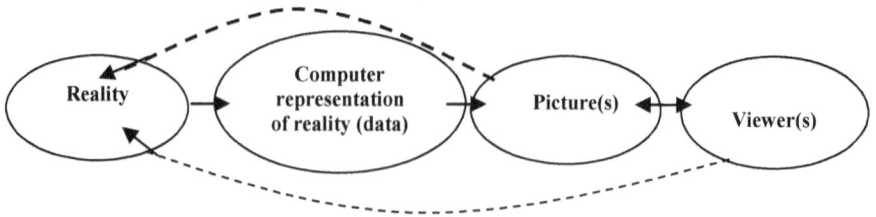

*It is critical that when you start the Lifestyle Challenges and throughout the 21 days (non-stop) and thereafter you establish a new pattern in your brain by focusing on and repeating the following thought processes. Remember that your mind has accepted how you are today because of your vision. Your personal picture never had the opportunity to change until now.

Lifestyle Challenge 3
Visualisation (Mental imagery)

Program the non conscious part of your mind and see yourself in your mind's eye - not as you are now but how you would ideally like to be. If you do this on a daily basis and for a minimum of 21 days (non-stop), this will become an automatic process. To make it easier, picture it as putting new grooves on a record by replacing the old (negative) grooves with a view that, in time, your old negative thoughts will be taken over by brand new positive ones. For ease, find pictures from magazines or books of what you would like to look like and place them somewhere you can see them on a daily basis. If you have a computer, shrink or enlarge them and print them off and carry them everywhere with you. Place them wherever you can see them but remember, do not move on until you have done this. You will be well on your way to success once you have prepared your mind because your body will want to follow.

Set whatever goals you choose

The act of setting a worthy goal for something you have always wanted and reaching it through determination, discipline and hard work, changes the very fibre of your being and you become a stronger person, not just physically but also mentally and emotionally. Goals are very important with everything you desire in life, especially weight loss and if they are written down then this will be a bench mark for you to aim for. The most important part, as mentioned previously, is the start date because nothing else can or should take place before this has been established. The only person that can set this date is you. You have to know that when you begin there can be no distractions from friends, family or anything around you for 21 days (non-stop). There can be no reasons or openings for excuses, so choose the date wisely because you don't get what you want in life, you get what you deserve.

If you want success and achievement, if you want to lose weight, improve your health and transform your body, then set your goals and just go for it!

Lifestyle Challenge 4

WEIGHT LOSS GOALS

Start Date: _____

My long-term weight loss goal is to lose _____ by_____

My short-term weight loss goals are to lose:

1. _____ by_____ and
2. _____ by_____ and
3. _____ by_____

I plan to achieve my goals through these specific actions:

_____
_____
_____

The rewards for reaching my goals are:

1. _____ and
2. _____ and
3. _____

Signature: _____

All of these new behaviours will move you mentally and physically towards whatever you have been thinking about and focusing on, so you need to make sure your thoughts are all related to where you want to be and how you want to feel and look. Your inner mind must change first and the rest will follow suit.

Let us recap on what you have achieved so far:

- You should have written 10 reasons why you want to lose weight;

- You should have written 10 positive self-talk phrases;

- You should visualise how you want to look and feel as if you already have success and

- You should prepare to set realistic goals for your weight loss journey.

You can set your goals once you have read the book and then you can make them realistic and suited to you personally because at this stage you don't know what specific actions you can do, but soon you will.

Points to note before you choose this plan

In 1992 the British Heart Foundation was sufficiently concerned about dieting and how it increased the risk of heart disease, so much so that they produced and distributed a booklet alerting Doctors to the danger.

In addition to coronary disease and heart attacks, there are a number of other health problems associated with yo-yo dieting. These include the previously mentioned decrease in lean tissue (including heart muscle), loss of bone minerals, gout or gallstones, hair loss, fibrosis and tissue scarring, high blood pressure when returning to a normal diet, depression, harmful side effects of appetite depressant drugs, and shortened lifespan.

Points to note:

- There is no "magic bullet" when it comes to nutrition and there isn't one single diet that works for every person so you need to find an eating plan that works for you;

- Good nutrition doesn't come in a vitamin supplement and you should only take a vitamin with your doctor's recommendation because your body benefits the most when you eat healthy foods;

- Eating all different kinds of foods is best for your body. So learn to try new foods;

- Fad diets offer short term changes, but good health comes from long term effort and commitment;

- Stories from people who have used a diet program or product, especially in commercials and infomercials are advertisements; these people are usually paid to endorse what the ad is selling;

- Remember, regained weight or other problems that develop after someone has completed the diet program are never talked about in adverts and

- Filling our plates with the right food will, over time, eliminate obesity and dramatically reduce the incidence of self inflicted diseases associated with poor diet (Packer and Colman, 1999).

What choices are already out there

Meal replacements:
These are usually in the form of milkshakes, biscuits, snack bars and even chocolate and they are potentially extremely dangerous. Apart from doing nothing to encourage healthier, long term eating habits, they may not provide all the nutrients you require and could therefore lead to malnutrition and excessive weight loss, the dangers of which have already been noted.

Ready meals:
In May of 1992, Food magazine analysed popular calorie-counted ready meals promoted as slimming aids. They found that they were all lacking in fibre and healthy fats.

Pills:
At present, 12-17 million people are hooked on diet pills and the figures are rising. But we are ultimately talking about a $1.25 billion industry for fat absorbing pills (just one type). That's a lot of money for something that doesn't supply you with the solution and increases damage, not just within your body, but also within your mind. There are also products that you take before meals to fill you up and reduce your appetite and these are also usually in tablet form. These may cause wind or constipation, not to mention giving you no solution to your problem.

Surgery:
An increasingly large number of people are turning to surgery with an attitude of "If all else fails, cut it off or suck it out." Liposuction, perhaps the most common surgery, quite literally sucks out fat from under the skin and has seen a number of cases of post operative pain, infection and disfigurement. The fat sometimes grows back in lumps and middle-aged and older people may be left with flabby, sagging skin. There is also the additional risk of blood clots, permanent numbness in the area, severe bruising, loss of blood and lowered immunity to infection. Besides, it can't be good to suck out fat from inside the belly without the risk of damaging internal organs.
Bypass surgery or gastric banding limits the amount of food you can take in and some operations also restrict the amount of food you can digest. Many people have this type of surgery to lose weight quickly but, if you follow diet and exercise recommendations, you can keep the majority of the weight off. The surgery option however has risks and complications, including infections, hernias and blood clots.

Diet plan only:
Permanent or temporary weight loss, which will your new diet achieve? It's often easier, for short term results, to make drastic changes to your diet, although it seems to be counterintuitive because starting a whole new eating plan tends to make things simple in the early days of a diet. You might hate the food and feel hungry but you know exactly what you can and can't eat and, if you follow the diet, you'll lose weight, simple as that. No decisions, no choices, no room for mistakes. Why then would I persuade people not to do that?

The reason is in the length of time such a solution lasts because most people have given up a drastic plan like this within a week or two, especially in January with New Year's resolutions. Either they can't get the ingredients one day or they hate the food. They were too hungry, they had a night out and couldn't eat according to the plan and went completely off the rails.

Even if you manage to stick to the plan, what happens at the end of it after you lose weight? The problem is you have learned nothing new, you are right back where you were with your old habits and eating just as much as you always did. The weight comes right back as mentioned before, the classic yo-yo situation.

The way to achieve permanent weight loss is to make permanent adjustments to your diet and habits, ones that you are happy to live with for the rest of your life and, let's face it, the Lifestyle Challenges haven't been that difficult so far have they? It's not as easy as the drastic diet plan until you get into the swing of making those changes but, within a minimum of 21 days or so, they will become new habits and then they will become very easy indeed. What's more, those changes will remain with you forever and the weight will be gone for good.

On the following page is one of the best choices I have found for you and it is an example of a typical day of 2400 calories for someone who is not doing any physical training. Later in the book there is another example of a typical day of 2400 calories for someone who is doing physical training. These examples are both from Mike Geary, author of Truth about Abs.

Meals	Prot (g)	Carbs (g)	Fat (g)	Cals (g)	Fibre (g)
Breakfast					
1 cup fibre cereal (at least 5 - 6g /serving) 1 cup skimmed or raw milk, 5-6 sliced strawberries	14	64	1	300	7
2 whole eggs any style, 1 slice cheese	16	0	13	181	0
Water or unsweetened iced tea					
Mid morning meal					
¾ cup cottage cheese mixed with ¾ cup vanilla yoghurt, ¼ cup fibre cereal, ½ cup frozen berries and ¼ cup slivered almonds.	37	46	16	446	10
Water or unsweetened iced tea					
Early afternoon meal					
Whole wheat wrap with 1/5 lb chicken breast, diced avocado, salsa, lettuce, little cheese.	30	30	12	330	6
1 piece fruit (apple, orange, pear etc)	1	23	0	84	4
Water or unsweetened iced tea					
Late afternoon meal					
2 tbsp peanut butter on 1 slice whole grain bread, topped with fresh berries	12	25	16	274	6
1 cup skimmed milk	8	12	0	80	0
Dinner					
¼ lb lean organic meat (eye round steak, chicken breast, pork tenderloin, fish etc)	26	0	5	149	0
½ large sweet potato with little butter, cinnamon	2	29	5	160	3
Steamed vegetables (unlimited)	2	8	0	34	2
Mixed green salad with 1 tbsp extra virgin oil and 1 – 2 tbsp balsamic vinegar	1	10	14	164	2
Water					
Late night snack					
1/2 cup 1% cottage cheese with pineapple and ¼ cup coconut milk mixed in.	16	20	11	237	2
Totals for day	165	267	93	2439	42

Macronutrient Profile (Fibre excluded from calorie count)
Prot = Protein 27.1%
Carbs = Carbohydrates 38.6%
Fat 34.3%

Follow a similar diet to the one above for 6 days/week; then have one relaxed day. In the next chapter, the details about nutrition and how it affects dieting will be exposed and how you can achieve long term weight loss from eating certain food types.

MAKING SENSE OF ALL THE DIFFERENT FOODS OUT THERE

"One often learns more from ten days of agony than from ten years of contentment."

- Merle Shain

Balancing the figures

Before today, you must have seen a "healthy eating pyramid," a diagram that indicates the foods that you should eat more of and vice versa. I have created one of my own, especially for you, and you'll discover that as you read through the book eating the right balance of carbohydrates, fats and proteins to include a variety of fresh fruits, vegetables and whole grains, will supply your body with the vitamins, minerals, phyto-nutrients and fibre it needs. Sticking to these basic rules is recommended in order to not only weight loss but also to look after your health as a whole.

Below is an example of one way that you can get your daily calories:

40 - 50%
The percentage of your daily calories should come from good carbohydrates (beans, whole grains, berries etc). The majority should come from less-refined, unprocessed foods with a low to moderate Glycaemic load (GL). The GL ranks how quickly the body converts food to blood sugar, which can cause greater fluctuations in insulin le-vels and result in health problems. This will be explained in more detail later in this chapter.

30%
The percentage of your daily calories that should come from healthy fats, mainly mo-nounsaturated (good sources include olive oil, nuts, avocados, etc.) and omega-3s (flaxseeds, fortified eggs, walnuts, or fish, such as salmon and sardines).

20 – 30%
The percentage of your daily calories that should come from healthy lean protein sources, such as chicken, fish, reduced-fat dairy products and especially soybeans and soy foods.
As you can see in this example, it is suggesting that you consume a higher percentage of fat than protein. This is because there are a number of healthy fats that our bodies need and this will be reiterated later in the chapter.

Learn about carbohydrates in more detail

The carbohydrate (sugars, starches, and fibres') is the main source of energy for the human body. It is also the fuel that we need so that every cell in our body works effec-tively and efficiently.

One (1) gram of carbohydrate is equal to four (4) calories.

In our homes we have a carbohydrate choice, which can be compared to the choice we make when we decide which fuel to put in our cars. With carbohydrates it's either sim-ple or complex. When you eat food your digestive system breaks down starches and sugars into glucose that is used to create usable high powered energy for your body. Fibre, however, is not broken down. It acts as the body's cleanser and the soluble (wa-ter absorbent) fibre found in beans and many whole grains may help lower LDL (bad) cholesterol and blood pressure and reduce the risk of heart disease, diabetes, and some cancers. Carbohydrates such as fibres' and starches are known as complex and carbohydrates such as sugars are known as simple. In their natural state, all carbohydrates are great. Nature blends the simple and the complex and adds essential micro-nutrients for proper digestion and utilization of all the carbohydrates, proteins, and fat.

Carbohydrates are considered simple or complex based upon their chemical structure. Both types contain four calories per gram and both are digested into the bloodstream as glucose, which is then used to fuel our bodies for normal daily activity and exercise. The main differences between simple and complex carbohydrates are explained below:

Simple carbohydrates or simple sugars - The body breaks down and quickly absorbs these foods. This process causes a spike in insulin and, over time, this pattern can cause insulin resistance in some people. But most simple carbohydrates contain refined sugars and very few essential vitamins and minerals. Examples include table sugar, fruit juice, milk, yoghurt, honey, molasses, maple syrup and brown sugar. "The real villain is the food manufacturing industry," says Michael Van Straten, author of Super Energy Detox.
He goes on to talk about the sugar in processed foods and how people become accustomed to the 'sugar trap' in foods like:

- Desserts such as ice cream;

- Juices/canned drinks;

- Sugar coated breakfast cereals and

- Biscuits/sweets.

He says that "Once you have acquired a sweet tooth, its not long before every cup of tea or coffee needs three heaped spoons of sugar and every unoccupied moment is filled with a biscuit, a piece of cake or a Danish pastry."

Complex carbohydrates - Complex carbohydrates, however, take longer to digest and don't cause that spike in blood sugar. So insulin is therefore released in a more desirable, gradual manner and is packed with fibre, vitamins and minerals. Examples include vegetables, whole grain breads, oatmeal, legumes, brown rice and whole wheat pasta.

A study, published in the American Journal of Clinical Nutrition, showed that people who added whole grains, such as whole oats and whole-wheat bread, to their diets lost more weight. Researcher Pauline Koh-Banerjee, ScD, and her colleagues at the Harvard School of Public Health studied 27,000 men aged between 40 and 75 years old and found that the more whole grains they ate, the more weight they lost while dieting. They said that "fibre in the diet may fill people up faster than processed grains and perhaps help to regulate blood sugar levels. Moreover, because of their high fibre and water content, whole-grain foods contain fewer calories gram forgram than does (the same) amount of corresponding refined grain food.

Eating 40 grams of whole grains a day cuts middle age weight gain by as much as 3.5 pounds. All it takes is about 1 cup of oatmeal, or 3/4 cup of brown rice, or several slices of brown bread each day."

Simple carbohydrates & weight loss

As valid research and better information is being presented to the public, people are learning that simple carbohydrate consumption can drastically hinder anyone trying to maintain or lose weight.

CJ Segal-Isaacson, assistant professor at the Albert Einstein School of Medicine, completed a CCARB (Controlled Carbohydrate Assessment Registry Bank) study that examined the physical activity and health patterns of 1,300 people over a three-year period. At the one-year point in her study, results showed that individuals controlling carbohydrates, eating an adequate amount of protein and increasing their intake of non-starchy, nutrient-dense vegetables have consistently maintained weight loss over the last 18 months. In addition, the CCARB study has shown in regression analysis that carbohydrate intake, fibre intake and frequency of workouts were strong predictors of weight change in the reported participants. Of the 34.5 percent of people in her study who have gained over five pounds in the last 18 months, simple carbohydrate consumption, such as added sugar, was the single biggest indicator of the weight gain.
It seems clear that consuming adequate protein sources, in addition to non-starchy vegetables like dark, leafy greens, and limiting carbohydrate intake can be a viable option for losing or maintaining weight as a long-term approach to eating. There is more on protein later in this chapter.

Understand the carbohydrate-restricted diet

Studies show that a carbohydrate-restricted diet results in a significant reduction in fat mass and an increase in lean body mass in normal-weight men, which may be partially mediated by the reduction in circulating insulin concentrations. There are however, disadvantages to this type of diet and they are as follows:

- For most people, strict low-carb diets are difficult to stick to;

- Very low-carb diets are often unbalanced and missing many nutrients;

- Very low-carb diets may cause low energy levels and

- The initial rapid weight loss on a very low-carb diet can be deceiving.

If you remove most of the carbohydrates from your diet for a long period of time, you're setting yourself up for a relapse. What you cannot have you tend to crave, both physiologically and psychologically. Therefore, the more you cut the carbs, the easier it is to rebound when you start eating carbs again. You will feel physically tired if carbohydrates are restricted from your diet and you will more than likely become mentally irritable. Your level of energy will be extremely low which, in turn, would equal zero results with your weight loss program.

A carbohydrate restricted diet would normally involve the removal of entire food groups, such as fruits and 100% whole natural grains, which is definitely not nutritionally balanced for fibre, phytochemical and micronutrient intake. All of these facts make low-carbohydrate diets a poor choice for people who need to get active in order to lose weight. On low-carbohydrate diets, water and even lean tissue are much of the initial weight loss. So, if you drop 5-7 lbs in your first week, it will of course sound very impressive. But if one pound is fat, 2-3 pounds are water and 2-3 pounds are muscle, what did you accomplish? Your goal should be fat loss, not "weight" loss.

The few studies that have examined body composition after a carbohydrate-restricted diet have reported enhanced fat loss and preservation of lean body mass in obese individuals. A 6-week study conducted by Volek JS, Human Performance Laboratory, Department of Kinesiology, University of Connecticut, reported that fat mass was significantly decreased and approximately 70% of the variability in fat loss on the carbohydrate-restricted diet was accounted for by the decrease in insulin concentrations.

Discover the Glycaemic index

The Glycaemic index (GI) is a way of calculating the rate at which carbohydrate foods are digested and converted into sugar by the body. The lower the foods GI, the longer it takes for that food to be converted into sugar. By mixing these foods into a meal, a more even level of blood sugar will be able to be maintained. Using the GI can be a great help in planning a healthy diet that will provide you with a gradual release of energy and in doing so, help you avoid the sugar trap. Weight-loss diets may be more effective when dieters seek to reduce Glycaemic load (i.e. the amount their blood glucose rises after a meal) rather than limit fat intake. The findings indicate that a low Glycaemic diet may overcome the body's natural tendency to slow metabolism and turn on hunger cues to "make up" the missing calories.

Low Glycaemic Load (Low GL) diet
The low-Glycaemic load (low GL) diet reduces carbohydrates that are rapidly digested and raise blood sugar and insulin to high levels. Some of the foods include:

- White bread;

- Refined breakfast cereals and

- Concentrated sugars.

Instead, the low-Glycaemic load diet emphasises carbohydrates that release sugar more slowly, including whole grains, most fruits, vegetables, nuts, and legumes. Dr. David Ludwig, director of the Optimal Weight for Life (OWL), suggests that "the type of calories consumed, independent of the amount, can alter metabolic rate."

He goes on to say, "Almost anyone can lose weight in the short term, very few keep it off in the long term. That's given rise to the notion that the body has a 'set point' and that when you diet, internal mechanisms work to restore your weight to that set point. A low Glycaemic load (GL) diet, may work better with these internal biological responses to create the greatest likelihood of long term weight loss."

Below is an example of the difference between high and low Glycaemic load foods. The figures bracketed in the right hand column dictate slow digestion which means that once eaten, you'll be less hungry later.

Later in the book there is a shopping list for you that has been put together for slow burners. It's been added to assist you in buying the right foods.

OLD FAVORITES *(High Glycaemic load)*	BETTER BETS (Low Glycaemic load)
Breakfast	**Breakfast**
Bagel, white, frozen, 70g *(25)* Instant Cream of Wheat, 250g *(22)* Cornflakes, 30g *(21)* Grapefruit juice, 250g *(11)*	100% whole-grain bread, 30g (7) Oatmeal, 250g (13) All-bran cereal, 30g (4) Grapefruit, 120g (3)
Lunch	**Lunch**
Macaroni and cheese, 180g (32) Cranberry-juice cocktail, 250g (24) White rice, 150g (23) Corn chips, 50g (17)	Fettuccini, 180g *(18)* Club soda, 250g *(0)* Brown rice, 150g *(18)* Popcorn, 20g (8)
Dinner	**Dinner**
White spaghetti, 180g (27) Baked russet potatoes, 150g (26) Vanilla cake, frosting, 111g (24) Fanta Orange soft drink, 250g (23)	Whole-wheat spaghetti, 180g *(16)* Baked beans, 150g *(7)* Banana cake, no sugar, 80g *(16)* Unsweetened apple juice *(12)*

Protein and weight loss revealed

Proteins are molecules made up of amino acids, which the body breaks down and absorbs in order to rebuild and repair tissues. Humans need about 20 amino acids in order to live but our bodies can make most of them on their own. One (1) gram of protein is equal to four (4) calories.

As with low carbohydrate diets, there have been studies to show the effect of protein in weight loss. Skov AR from the Research Department of Human Nutrition in Denmark studied the effect on weight loss in obese subjects by the replacement of carbohydrate by protein. It was a study over six months with 65 healthy subjects involved, a mixture of overweight and obese people, 50 of them women and 15 of them men, all aged between 18-55 years.

The weight loss after six months was:

- 5.1 kg in the high-carbohydrate group.

- 8.9 kg in the high-protein group.

- Fat loss was 4.3 kg and 7.6 kg, respectively.

- No changes occurred in the control group

Replacement of some dietary carbohydrate by protein improves weight loss and increases the proportion of subjects achieving a clinically relevant weight loss.

This study also demonstrates that increasing the proportion of protein to carbohydrate in the diet has positive effects on body composition, blood lipids, glucose homeostasis and satiety during weight loss.

All you need to know about fat loss and weight loss

Not fearing the fats
From a health point of view, most people in the western world would benefit from reducing their fat intake but reducing to very low levels can be harmful. We need fat for the provision of essential fatty acids and the provision and absorption of fat-soluble vitamins. Good fats, like omega-3 fatty acids, which the body can't produce on its own, help with brain function and children's development, and they may stave off heart disease and arthritis. One gram of fat is equal to nine (9) calories and therefore it stands to reason that a low fat diet will assist in weight loss due to an intake of reduced calories.

Current scientific evidence indicates that dietary fat plays a role in weight loss and maintenance such as the CARMEN study that was completed at the Nutrition and Toxicology Research Institute in the Netherlands by Saris WH, who investigated the long term effects of changes in dietary carbohydrate/fat ratio and simple versus complex carbohydrates.

A total of 398 moderately obese adults took part in the study over a period of six (6) months and were divided into two (2) main groups:

- A low fat, high simple carbohydrate group and

- A low fat, high complex carbohydrate group

The findings suggested that reduction of fat intake results in a modest but significant reduction in body weight and body fatness. The increase in either simple or complex carbohydrates did not indicate significant differences in weight change. These findings underline the importance of this dietary change and its potential impact on the public health implications of obesity.

How excess body fat can affect your body

Scientists have long known that overweight people have increased inflammation levels but they now believe that at least some of this inflammation can be traced back to the fat itself. In people who are overweight or obese, fat cells churn out proteins known as cytokines, which can induce low grade systemic inflammation. A lot of refined vegetable oils such as corn and safflower are high in omega-6s which are pro-inflammatory. Adding that low level inflammation may contribute to disease, when it comes to excess body fat, location is critical. The greatest source of inflammation is the fat around our abdomen. For your information, blueberries, cherries, and blackberries are rich in anti-inflammatory flavonoid compounds.

A study was completed at the Research Department of Human Nutrition & LMC in Denmark by Astrup A. and colleagues. They studied the role of dietary fat in body fatness.

The study concluded that:

- A low fat diet, high in protein and fibre rich carbohydrates, mainly from different vegetables, fruits and whole grains, is highly satiating for fewer calories than fatty foods and

- This diet composition provides good sources of vitamins, minerals, trace elements and fibre and may have the most beneficial effect on blood lipids and blood pressure levels.

A reduction in dietary fat without restriction of total energy intake prevents weight gain in subjects of normal weight and produces a weight loss in overweight subjects, which is highly relevant for public health.

In the next chapter some cures for compulsive eating and food cravings will be revealed to you and you will discover how to manage stress.

DISCOVER CURES FOR COMPULSIVE EATING AND FOOD CRAVINGS

"The real act of discovery is not in finding new lands but in seeing with new eyes."

- Marcel Proust

Stress and its relationship with weight gain

Physiologically speaking, you react to everyday stresses in ways that make junk food, like chocolate bars, cookies and chips, all the more tempting. Take the supermarket scenario from the crying baby to the fact that you're late, your agitation increases the longer you stand in line. Your body responds by releasing a stress hormone called cortisol, which, in turn, triggers the release of neuropeptide and galanin (two neurotransmitters). These are chemicals within the brain that affect your mood, keep you alert and boost your energy.

They also make you increasingly hungry for sugary and fatty foods. At the same time as this is happening, cortisol the stress hormone, is released and suppresses serotonin, a calming neurotransmitter that helps keep depression and anxiety under control. As you can imagine, all of these biological factors make healthy eating that much more difficult.

Start your stress less eating plan with:

- A gradual reduction of processed foods;

- Consuming a reduced amount of refined carbohydrates, as these rank among the greatest stress culprits and

- Limit, or even better still, eliminate fast foods as the trans-fatty acids that most fast foods contain actually reduce circulation and raise blood pressure, keeping your body in a constant state of stress.

We already know about sugar and sweet food choices and the implications that they have on the body. We need to cut them from our diets because they raise insulin levels too high and, although sugar increases serotonin that keeps depression and anxiety under control, it's only temporary. Therefore, they take our moods up and then they crash right back down again.

The best thing is prevention. Keep healthy options ready for when you're bored. For example, stash fresh fruit or unsalted cashews in your bag for a quick fix. Get rid of all temptations from the house/ office drawer/ glove compartment and anywhere else they may entice you.

How you can manage stress

These days I'm sure you rarely get the chance to relax and studies show that 90 percent of all illnesses, both mental and physical, are related to stress. Therefore, anything you do to dampen that physiological response can help your health.

The secret to success is to chill out in stages, grabbing a bit of focused relaxation when you can. Research shows that people who can go somewhere quiet and relax for just 20 minutes, a couple of times a day, are half as likely to be admitted to a hospital.

Scientifically, exercise has been shown to reduce levels of stress hormones but remember that any activity that relaxes you counts as a stress reducer. If all else fails, a stress-reducing supplement called Holy Basil (available at most health food stores) is a great example of an adaptogen, which helps your body cope with stress and manage cortisol levels. Please note that Holy Basil is not recommended for women who are pregnant or trying to conceive.

Below is a table to assist you:

STRESS FIGHTERS	HELPFUL NUTRIENT	WHY IT HELPS
Avocados, baked potatoes (with skin), bananas, chickpeas, yellow-fin tuna	Vitamin B6	Stress depletes B6, which helps produce serotonin, a calming neurotransmitter.
Clams, milk (fat-free), plain yoghurt (fat-free), salmon, sardines	Vitamin B12	Along with other B vitamins, B12 helps form GABA, a calming neurotransmitter.
Asparagus, chickpeas, lentils, oatmeal, orange juice	Folate (folic acid)	Folic acid helps make dopamine, a neurotransmitter associated with pleasure.
Almonds, amaranth, spinach, sunflower seeds, tofu, wild rice	Magnesium	Stress depletes magnesium, which stimulates the production of GABA and helps make dopamine.
Broccoli, brussel sprouts, orange juice, red and green peppers, strawberries	Vitamin C	Vitamin C boosts your immune system and fights brain-cell damage resulting from constant exposure to cortisol.

Do you get enough sleep?

A lack of zzz's impairs your body's ability to heal itself and lowers brain function. Studies have shown that a person who gets only five hours of sleep can exhibit the motor skills of someone who has drank two alcoholic beverages. Staying up late also screws up cortisol levels, putting you more at risk for diabetes and obesity.

Secrets to success:

- Try to hit the sack by 10 p.m. and get eight hours of rest. If you go to bed at 10 and wake up by 6, your body will get its optimal levels of healthy hormone fluctuations. If you can't make it to bed by 10, then go to bed by midnight and get up at 8;

- If you're a night owl, naturally train your body by going to bed 15 minutes earlier each week. If you toss and turn once you're under the covers, don't self-medicate with over the counter remedies, which can leave you with a morning hangover effect;

- Dim the lights a half an hour before bedtime and turn down the heat. Low light signals your brain that it's time to sleep and cooler air promotes the small body temperature drop that occurs when you slumber and

- If all else fails and you don't get your eight hours, make it up by napping. A 15-minute nap can make you feel infinitely better, although anything longer than about 20 minutes can be too much of a good thing because if it's too long or too late in the day it can interfere with your night time sleep.

Melatonin, our sleep hormone, spikes between midnight and 1a.m., so you don't want to be awake then. It's a very powerful antioxidant and anti-inflammatory and it decreases the amount of oestrogen your body produces and it stimulates your immune system.

Your seven cures for compulsive eating and food cravings

Although you should not forbid yourself food, you can get rid of cravings by actually eating small amounts of the food in a controlled way. But there may be times when you just want to eat treat after treat and, as you know, eating too many unplanned treats will wreck your weight loss attempts. So how do you cope with that? Several studies have demonstrated that eating low energy dense foods, such as fruits, vegetables, and soups, maintains satiety while reducing energy intake. In a clinical trial advising individuals to eat portions of low energy dense foods was a more successful weight loss strategy than fat reduction coupled with restriction of portion sizes. Eating satisfying portions of low energy dense foods can help to enhance satiety and control hunger while restricting energy intake for weight (Ello-Martin, JA, 2005).

Here are a few things to do before you "give in" to an unplanned craving:

1. When you feel you want to eat something, have a glass of water or a cup of herbal or fruit tea. Maybe you were just thirsty and not really hungry at all. Drink something before you do anything else;

2. Get up and take a quick walk, even if it's just to another floor in your office building, or do a few stretches and remind yourself of your goals for your body;

3. Take your toothbrush and toothpaste with you everywhere. Go and brush your teeth, you won't want to lose that clean fresh feeling;

4. If you still really want the food, ask yourself if you are really hungry;

5. Analyze the situation and decide what has really tempted you. If you have a sudden urge to eat something, why was that? Did you see food on offer? Did you wander past the fridge? Did you suddenly feel bored with what you were doing? You may see that you don't really need the food, it was just an impulse;

6. Make a judgment and if you are physically hungry, think about what will really satisfy your hunger. Do you need something sweet, something crunchy, something to nibble, something salty or something to fill you up? There is usually something healthy that can satisfy any type of hunger. Keep substitutes available for unhealthy treats and

7. The bottom line is, if nothing else will do, have the food. Eat it slowly and enjoy it without guilt. You really wanted it. Now make up for it during the rest of the day with a little extra exercise here and a smaller portion there to get things back on track.

In the next chapter, 'Visualise the New You' will assist you in changing your attitude to food and help you to look at things more differently and for the better.

CHANGING YOUR ATTITUDE ABOUT FOOD

"Change your thoughts and you change your world."

- Norman Vincent Peale

42

Understand your physical and emotional reasons for food

Most people on a diet or a mission to lose weight get to a point where they hate food and wonder why it is controlling the way they look and feel. This attitude, of course, becomes one of resentment and an inner sadness, which clearly affects the emotional state of each individual.

Physical reasons:

- Not eating enough volume of food which leaves you with an empty tummy too soon after a meal;

- Not eating enough calories, leaving you with low blood sugar and a need to eat pretty quickly to correct it and

- Eating foods that are high in fast releasing carbohydrate or sugar (high GI foods), which give a spike to your blood sugar and a rapid decline as your body tries to correct it.

Emotional reasons:

- Delicious foods are all around you, making it difficult to resist;

- Feeling down and eating for comfort;

- Eating to plug a gap inside because you literally feel 'empty' and

- Eating because you are bored, which is the case with many people who are hungry all the time, as eating literally passes the time.

Life is sweeter without refined sweets but when you are stressed you will eat sweeter, fatty foods and you will ultimately increase your appetite for carbohydrates and fat.

Eat your way to a better attitude

To achieve a constant energy balance and a healthy weight, you must aim to limit your energy intake from total fats and shift fat consumption away from the worst of the saturated fats to unsaturated fats and towards the elimination of trans-fatty acids. You should try to increase your consumption of fruits, vegetables, whole grains and nuts but most of your efforts should be to focus on limiting your intake of free sugars and salt from all sources and ensure that if you have to have salt, it is iodized.

Fill up on fibre

As mentioned previously, incorporate beans, legumes, and whole grains, such as brown rice or quinoa, into your diet. Also, try and add nuts into your diet by sprinkling almonds, hazelnuts or walnuts on cereal or salads or stash them in your desk drawer for a healthy alternative to vending machine rubbish.

Fine tune your fats
Sort out your kitchen and get rid of most saturated fats and all trans-fats by avoiding margarine and anything with hydrogenated oil in it. Replace them with healthier options, such as extra virgin olive oil and flaxseed oil.

Eat more plant & fish based proteins
If you eat a lot of red meat you should attempt to at least substitute it with soy or fish a few times a week because animal proteins contain arachidonic acid, which the body uses to produce pro-inflammatory prostaglandins. Wild salmon, sardines and herring are rich in omega-3 fats and relatively low in the toxin mercury. Attempt to look out for the "Seafood Safe" label or, if in doubt, consider taking a fish-oil supplement.

Attitude to water
Staying hydrated is the best way to:

- Flush out toxins from the body;

- Ease digestion;

- Maintain energy and

- Promote good brain function and all around health.

Think of water as a health boosting beverage and if you want to feel less bloated and leaner, you need to avoid all soda drinks. As for diet sodas with sugar substitutes, they just stimulate a craving for more sweetness. Most people need a coffee in the morning but too much caffeine jacks up your body and confuses your hunger signals. If you work in an office, take in your water and see how better you feel. One week you will have a small bottle on your desk and a month or so later, if not before, you will have a 1.5 litre bottle under your desk…you'll see!

When you feel thirsty, the only liquids you should drink are water or herbal tea because anything caffeinated is a diuretic. Instead, try to drink 100 ounces of water a day. Try filling a 32-ounce container and keep track of how often you have to refill it. Once you've emptied it three times, you've almost hit your target. Aim to empty the first bottle by 10 a.m., the next by 1 p.m., and the last by late afternoon. If regular water bores you, add a slice of lemon or cucumber to your glass (just like at the spa), or try a flavoured, calorie free water.

Attitude to vitamins
Are you getting all your essential nutrients? Believe it or not, 99 out of 100 Americans don't even come close to meeting the minimum standards. Even small vitamin and mineral deficiencies that you have today can lead to big time health problems, such as osteoporosis, tomorrow.

Vitamin-C status is inversely related to body mass. Individuals with adequate vitamin-C status oxidize 30% more fat during a moderate exercise bout than individuals with low vitamin-C status. Therefore, vitamin-C depleted individuals may be more resistant to fat mass loss (Johnston, CS, 2005).

Four secrets to vitamin success:

1. Supplements ensure you are covered in case you don't get everything you need from food;

2. If you're female, you probably need calcium and vitamin D;

3. If you're menstruating, you need a multivitamin with iron and

4. If you're vegetarian, you most definitely need iron but a multivitamin alone often won't cut it because iron and calcium can't be given in the same pill as they bind to each other, decreasing absorption.

How you take a supplement also matters:

- You must have food in your stomach in order to absorb nutrients, but it's not necessarily as easy as tossing back your pills right after breakfast;

- The compounds in coffee and tea, whether it's regular or decaf coffee or black or herbal tea, will block iron absorption, so don't take a supplement when those are in your stomach;

- Citrus and vitamin-C, on the other hand, aid the absorption of vitamins, so it always helps to take your multivitamin with a little orange or grapefruit juice and

- Line your vitamins up next to your toothbrush, and take them with a small glass of juice before brushing your teeth at bedtime.

Attitude to calories
Our bodies can distinguish one type of calorie from another. We handle fat calories, carbohydrate calories and protein calories differently. Some tend to be stored as fat while some tend to be digested more quickly but knowing the distinction and eating accordingly can help ease blood-sugar woes and protect your health.

Attitude to fats
There are still people who believe that fat intake should be kept as low as possible but it's the kind of fats you eat that matters. We hear so much about saturated fat from doctors, nutritionists, fitness professionals, and the media. The fact about saturated fat being bad for us has actually never been proven and, although saturated fat intake does increase your LDL (bad cholesterol), it actually increases your HDL (good cholesterol) even further, hence improving your overall cholesterol ratio. Maybe we need to get our facts straight and figure out who we should be listening to.

Sugar, carbohydrates & Trans fats
Experts agree that these are the big three, the axis of evil that leaves us chubby and
cranky. Along with spiking insulin levels and packing on pounds, sugar inflames cells
and makes skin more sensitive to sun damage and premature aging. Beyond the way we
look and feel there's also our future health to consider. Women who have higher insulin
levels from consuming mass amounts of sugar also have a more than 280% higher risk
of developing breast cancer. Trans-fats promote inflammation and the production of
free radicals that contribute to chronic disorders like dementia, Alzheimer's, arthritis,
heart disease, cancer, premature aging, and the list only goes on.

Attitude to cholesterol
All over the world people have become aware of the dangers that cholesterol poses to
their health. The greatest risks target the heart, so much so that cholesterol has become
synonymous with fatal heart attacks. Of course, this is slightly exaggerated, though in
general medical terms, high cholesterol is one of the deadliest afflictions of the modern
world.

Attitude to organic foods
Certified organic produce is not essentially healthier than produce that has been grown
under non organic conditions and the nutritional content of a particular vegetable
doesn't change. But the lack of synthetic, pesticide residues on organically grown produce definitely makes for a safer product.

Attitude to whole grain
There is strong clinical evidence linking the consumption of whole grains to a reduced
risk of coronary heart disease (Anderson, 2002). With this disease being the number
one cause of death and disability in the USA, in both men and women I'd say that it
would be extremely wise to change our attitude towards whole grain foods.

Attitude to Glycaemic load (GL)
Glycaemic load (GL) is a measure of how quickly carbohydrates turn into sugar in your
body. When you pulverize starch into flour, it has a huge surface area for enzymes to
react on and turns quickly into sugar. High GL foods cause blood sugar to spike and
insulin secretion to surge, over time this pattern may lead to insulin resistance, obesity,
diabetes and other health problems.

Why you should shop for labels

In the grocery store is where your secret to success begins, especially if you eat at home on a regular basis. If you do, you must read package labels.

It would be wise to study the ingredients of foods advertised as:

- Low / non fat;

- Fat free;

- High protein;

- Low cholesterol / carbohydrates etc and

- Reduced sugar. Pass on any food that names sugar as one of its first three in-gredients, even if its sucrose, high fructose corn syrup, brown sugar, or honey as it's all sugar.

Dietary Components - Labels on foods have changed so much over the years but now the FDA and administrations like it have taken on the task of making the most sweeping changes to food labelling in a generation. Susan Thom, a registered dietician of Parma in Ohio, knows how important it is for people to know the number of calories from fat they eat each day. She states that "you need to limit fat consumption to 30 percent or less of total daily calories." But in the past, obtaining that information from the food label has required some mathematical skill, namely, multiplying the total grams (g) of fat in a serving by nine since 1g of fat contains nine calories. She also says that, "it does take time, but if you want to feed yourself well, you have to look at the label." For millions of people who seek to restrict their fat intake to recommended levels, a new dietary component has been added to the food label - 'calories from fat.'

Trans Fat

Whatever you do when you are out shopping and checking labels, you must reject anything with trans-fats, which may be listed as partially hydrogenated vegetable oils. Remember to crunch the numbers on the labels. If you buy a product like crackers and they claim to have zero trans-fats in them, look closer at the label. You may find that it has less than half a gram per serving, which might be listed as three crackers. Of course, when you eat three servings (i.e. nine crackers), you're getting too many trans-fats in your system.

In this case, the ingredient list reveals more than the nutrition label. A product can say zero trans-fats and still have a small percentage. How so? The FDA allows for up to half a gram of trans-fat under the "zero" label.

The Institute of Medicine, however, maintains that there's no safe minimum level of trans-fat. Look out for ingredients, such as shortening or partially hydrogenated oil, to tip you off that the food contains some trans-fat. If a food has just one gram or more of combined saturated and trans-fats per 100 calories, you must put it back and should aim to want to get your trans-fat consumption down to zero.

Colour of food

You should always consider a foods colour, especially in breads, rice and pasta made from whole grains, which are often brown. These are definitely what you need as they are digested more slowly than refined white ones. As you have read previously, the body processes white bread, rice and pasta as sugar almost immediately, causing insulin spikes. So if you endeavour (over a period of time) to replace every white food you eat with something brown, then you will definitely notice the difference.

Soy

We hear a lot about the benefits of soy but, as with most things, moderation in this particular case is paramount as you can definitely eat too much soy and the type of soy you eat matters greatly. It's desirable to eat moderate, regular portions of fermented soy foods, like Miso and tempeh, traditional foods whose health benefits have been shown in Asian population studies. But, when it comes to highly refined soy products, such as fractionated soy foods, Tofu, soy protein isolate or added soy isoflavones found in certain protein powders and energy bars, there's no comparable evidence for health benefits. Soy isoflavones may carry risks associated with thyroid dysfunction so it's best to stay away from them.

Organic labelling

Organic junk food is still junk food. Some foods sound healthier but with all the sugar and oil, they are just a disguised version of the same thing minus the pesticides. To be 100% sure, read the labels first and of course use common sense.

Whole grain labels

When you buy products labelled "whole grain," you may assume you're getting a healthy dose of fibre, which helps keep your digestive system running smoothly and reduces your risk of numerous diseases. But like "organic," terms like "whole grain" can be misleading on packaged foods so always check the fibre content. The FDA states that whole-grain foods should contain the three key ingredients of cereal grains:

- Bran - the fibre filled outer part of the kernel;

- Endosperm - the inner part and usually all that is left in most processed grains and

- The germ - the heart of the grain kernel.

Plus, these three ingredients need to be present in the same relative proportion as they exist naturally, a way to be sure that manufacturers do not add back small amounts of each ingredient to highly processed food and then call it whole grain. While these guidelines are aimed at food companies, Barbara Schneeman, director of the FDA's Centre for Food Safety and Applied Nutrition said "it's also very important for consumers to have consistent and uniform terminology for what consists of a whole grain."

Shopping list for slow burners

I have listed some foods overleaf for you so that you can use them as additions to your shopping list.

This list is by no means inclusive of all the ones you need in order to speed up your metabolism, but just try them out for yourself.

ANIMAL PROTEIN	VEGETABLES	FRUITS
HOOFED	**FIBROUS 3 - 5 A DAY**	**2 – 4 A DAY**
Beef (lean)	Bean sprouts	Apple
POULTRY	Beetroot	Apricot
Chicken	Broccoli	Banana
Eggs	Brussels	Cantaloupe
Turkey	Cabbage	Cherry
DAIRY	Carrots	Grapefruit
Low fat cheese	Celery	Honeydew melon
Low fat milk	Cucumbers	Orange
Low fat yoghurt	Green beans	Peach
SEAFOOD	Kale	Pear
Catfish	Lettuce	Plum
Cod	Okra	
Flounder	Onions	
Haddock	Peppers	
Perch	Spinach	
Scrod	**STARCHY**	
Sole	Potato	
Swordfish	Squash	
Tuna	Yam	
Turbot		
VEGETABLE PROTEIN	**GRAINS & GRAIN PRODUCTS**	**FATS & OILS**
Miso	Brown rice	Olive oil
Tempeh	Kasha	Sesame oil
	Oatmeal	Canola oil
	Berries	Quinoa
		Butter
	BEVERAGES	
Water (approx. 2L or x8 glasses)	Herbal or any flavoured tea	Any blended vegetable juice or fruit juice using the above foods

Which beverages should you choose?

The beverages listed at the bottom of the shopping list (overleaf) are your best bet for weight loss and you should try as much as you can to avoid the following:

Slim fast shakes
Which are full of:

- Many chemicals;

- Hydrogenated oils and

- Fructose corn syrup.

Attempt to blend your own using skimmed milk, egg and any fruit you like, especially fresh or frozen berries.

Soda
Soda is a carbonated cocktail full of nasty chemicals and gut fattening high fructose corn syrup. This is the most evil thing you can put in your body and causes a myriad of health problems.

Diet sodas are full of artificial sweeteners which:

- Create a negative hormonal response;

- Increase fat storing hormones and

- Increase cravings for sweets and refined carbohydrates.

Cost
The manufacturers of junk foods would love for you to think that healthier options are more expensive but if you shop wisely, you'll see that some of the healthier food options don't cost that much more, if at all. In general, the less packaging, the less you'll pay and you will find that if you venture into a health food store and compare, you will be surprised by how inexpensive the foods are.
Bargains are also found at farmers markets because there's no middle man and of course, a reduced transport cost. Most processed foods are downright cheap but you must consider why?

The reason is because many are made with government subsidised ingredients, like corn oil and high fructose corn syrup. Even if they're inexpensive on the shelves, they're no bargain health wise. According to OZ Garcia, author of The Balance, "Certain foods speed up a sluggish metabolism, give you more energy and build up your resistance to diseases to which you may otherwise be prone."

Discover ways to cook & eat healthily at home

In this day and age we have become accustomed to and have allowed ourselves to become limited for time, which is usually because of our poor planning. Because of this, we tend to opt for easy solutions. For example, a drive-thru meal or some form of fast food. If we are at work for lunch, what we should do is prepare something the night before or simply choose a healthier option from all of the choices that are available.

If we can train our mind in this way, it will help solve many issues. When cooking at home, we should always fuel our bodies with foods that are steamed, garden fresh, boiled, baked, roasted, poached, lightly sautéed, or stir-fried but always avoid frying at all costs.

Below are some tips to get you on your way:

Snacks, ready to go
You probably have tons of tempting goodies lying around the house and most people feel the need to fill their houses with chocolate and cookies. Psychologically you know they are there and you'll be tempted when you get the slightest bit hungry. To counteract this you need to make sure that you have a ready to grab alternative in a plastic bag or box and filled with ready washed, peeled and chopped fruit and vegetables that you can pick at or can take with you wherever you go.

Oils
In the kitchen, use extra-virgin olive oil for dressings and low-heat dishes and use grape seed or expeller pressed organic canola oil for high-heat cooking. When it comes to anything generic like vegetable oil, there really is no telling what's inside, so it's best to steer clear of them at all costs.

Salad with everything
Eat a large side salad or a pile of vegetables with every meal and if you add this to the plate first then that just leaves half a plate left for the more calorie filled part of the meal.

Spices
Certain spices, such as ginger, garlic, onion, tumeric and rosemary, have strong anti inflammatory effects so make them an integral part of your diet. Try using ginger, garlic and onion in stir-fries, turmeric in soups and rosemary on roasted vegetables. Chilli is also awesome for weight loss.

Herbs
Throw out all old herbs and make a pledge to use only the freshest herbs. If you buy fresh herbs, they add so much flavour and complexity to food.

Grains
As mentioned before, go for actual grains instead of flour based foods as often as possible, simply because grains tend to have a lower Glycaemic load (GL). This doesn't

render bread off limits but try and pay close attention to the texture. For example, if you see big pieces of grain, that's a good sign that it has a lower GL. As for pasta, Italian whole wheat and Japanese soba are highly recommended. Some of the more familiar products that qualify as whole grains under the new definition include oatmeal, popcorn, shredded wheat and brown rice as well as barley, buckwheat, bulgur, wild rice, whole rye and the more exotic amaranth and quinoa.

Fish

Although it contains an important type of oil, fish is generally low in fat, which makes it a good food for maintaining a healthy weight. The healthiest way to cook fish is to steam, grill, bake and barbecue or microwave it.

However, it is okay to cook fish in a small amount of oil, such as olive, canola or peanut oil. Fish that is deep fried and battered is very high in fat. The same goes for fish cakes, fish fingers and fish served with rich, creamy sauces.

Meat

We now know that protein will fill us up and make us feel more satisfied during and after a meal. Therefore, chicken and turkey would be the healthiest choices and luckily there are endless ways that you can enjoy them in your diet:

- In salad;

- Stir fry;

- Curry and

- Sweet and sour dishes to name but a few

Know which meats are best

Below is a table of different meat choices and information so you will have more knowledge before you make your next meal.

MEAT	CONTENT	EXTRA INFORMATION	RECOMMENDATIONS
Bacon	Contains about 16g fat per 100g.	Is also very high in salt and usually contains nitrites which, once in the stomach, may form substances linked to cancer. Smoked foods also been implicated as having cancer-inducing potential.	Use bacon in small quantities, and eat only occasionally.
Beef	Contains about 5g of fat per 100g	About half this fat content is monounsaturated fat, similar to the fat found in heart-healthy olive oil.	If you buy minced (ground) beef, make sure it doesn't contain too much fat. The meat facts on beef show that it's fine to include from time-to-time in a healthy diet.

Chicken	Skinless chicken contains around 3g fat per 100g	If you're worried about calories, remove the skin, where most of the fat is found. Chicken is a good source of nutrients	Choose organic whenever you can, both to avoid supporting the battery farming industry and because the flavour is much better.
Duck	Contains 11g fat per 100g meat	Duck contains a lot more saturated fat than either chicken or turkey. It's a good source of iron & zinc.	Eat only occasionally and use in recipes where the skin is removed, such as stir fry's.
Ham	Contains about 3g fat per 100g	Also high in salt. The meat facts on ham don't make very pleasant reading. Packaged ham is often made from off cuts of pork which have been ground, reconstituted with water, starched to bind, then pressed and shaped into 'ham." This kind may be high in fat and additives.	Buy lean ham from a butcher or delicatessen, cut from a joint. Eat only in moderation.
Lamb	Contains around 8g fat per 100g	Lamb is quite fatty, particularly cuts like shoulder. But, as research continues, it's unclear just how harmful saturated fat is to the body.	Lamb is not often reared intensively and, in moderation, is a good addition to a healthy diet.
Offal	Liver and kidneys are lower in fat than meat and are nutritious foods	This is a definite case for buying organic, because the function of both the liver and kidneys is to detoxify the animal's body so they may contain harmful substances if the animal has been intensively reared.	Pregnant women are often advised to avoid liver because of its high vitamin A content, which could be harmful to the fetus.
Pork	Contains about 4g fat per 100g	The vast majority of pigs are intensively farmed so, there's a risk that their meat will contain chemicals such as antibiotics used in factory farming.	Look for organic or 'freedom' meats. These pigs are reared out of doors in communities and have freedom to roam.
Sausages	Contain around 25g fat per 100g	Mass-produced sausages are not only high in fat, they can also contain fillers, additives, lots of salt and mechanically retrieved meat.	Buy sausages from a farmer's market or reputable butcher, who should be using better quality ingredients. Eat only occasionally.
Turkey	Contains around 1g fat per 100g	Star of the meat facts list, turkey is one of the super foods and an excellent lean source of protein. It's also rich in B vitamins and zinc.	Buy organic.
Venison	Contains around 2.5g fat per 100g	Some venison is wild and some is farmed. But even when farmed, deer are seldom raised intensively.	Excellent healthy choice for those who like a robustly flavoured red meat.

If you eat red meat, select leaner cuts, like sirloin steak or filet mignon instead of most steaks, or pot roast instead of hamburgers or meat loaf. No matter what meal you're planning, strike a caloric balance of lean protein, healthy fats and complex carbohydrates. Together, these macro-nutrients stabilise your blood sugar, leaving you less likely to feel famished and desperate for that bag of chips. Your portions should be judged by the size of your fist because the size of your fist is identical to the size of your stomach. Therefore, if you eat more, your stomach has to stretch to consume what you are feeding it. Vegetables and fruits, however, can generally be consumed in large quantities because of their nutritious value. The US National Health and Nutrition Examinations Survey shows that sugar intake makes up 25% of total calories and fat intake approaches 34%, which means that foods that have poor nutritional value make up over half the daily calories.

Believe that eating out can be ok

For many people, restaurant dining is no longer reserved for special occasions, it's a daily event. However, that food will represent one third of all calories in the average diet. The nutrient content of restaurant meals is extremely difficult to assess and that became apparent when a survey conducted by researchers at New York University found that trained dieticians not only underestimated the calorie content of five restaurant meals by an average of 37%, they also underestimated fat content by 49%.

It will not always be possible for you to eat at home so plan ahead. If you are going out for the day with your children to a park, take along a healthy snack, such as an apple with some cheese, or if you are going to a cocktail party, eat before leaving home and avoid the heavy hors d'oeuvres. If you are going to a restaurant and it concerns you by not wanting to ruin your appetite, then carry a small bag of almonds on you. If you have a couple while walking to the restaurant for dinner, then it will prevent you from dipping into the bread and butter.

Your new restaurant tips

If you know what you're doing, it's relatively easy to keep your weight down while eating at restaurants, here are a few suggestions: Come up with a plan. You know what you like but decide what your priorities will be for that meal. If your choice is the fajitas, perhaps you can skip the rice and beans. If it's the cheesecake, order a light dinner, such as shrimp cocktail and salad with dressing on the side. Whatever happens, you should never be afraid to special order with the waiter because the chef will be happy to oblige. For example, if you really have your heart set on the special pasta dish with chicken, sun-dried tomatoes and mushrooms in a spicy cream sauce, consider these changes:

a) Ask the chef to sauté the chicken, tomatoes, and mushrooms in broth rather than oil

or

b) Ask the chef to use just half the cream sauce.

These small requests can result in a dish that is half the calories as the original and all it takes is for you to ask. Most restaurants want to please their customers and are usually willing to satisfy specific requests, such as the five below:

1. Order sauces and salad dressings on the side, or ask for low-calorie dressings;

2. Request salsa, mustard or flavoured vinegars to get fat free flavour;

3. Request half-portions at a reduced price or take home half the meal in a doggie bag;

4. Ask that foods be prepared with olive or canola oil instead of butter, margarine or shortening and

5. Request that foods be boiled or grilled instead of fried.

Eating in restaurants should be a fun experience but you should always stop eating when you are pleasantly full, not when your stomach is cursing at you. If you choose wisely, you can even leave without having to undo the top button of your jeans. If you do crave a dessert, opt for something low fat, like sorbet, fresh berries or fruit.

In the next chapter it will be revealed to you how certain ways to eat can affect your day, by just discovering when it is best to eat and how you should do it.

YOUR DAILY PURPOSE OF FOOD

"You must be the change you wish to see in the world."

- Gandhi

Purpose of food

Besides the growling in your stomach, there are several reasons to eat. You may be hungry because there was no nutritional value in your previous meal, you fill a plate to fill an emotional void or you're just plain bored. There is a purpose for food beyond the fact that it tastes good and provides a sensual pleasure for the palate and, if you don't eat, your biological mechanisms will fail, so it is a basic matter of survival. While searching for things that taste good, remember that the functions and mechanisms of your body thrive on whole food nutrition and, unfortunately, there is a very large gap between the dietary guidelines and what people actually eat. According to Nicola Reavley, author of Vitamins, Minerals, Supplements and herbs:

- On any one day, an estimated 45% of people don't consume any fruit or juice and 22% don't eat any vegetables. Less than 10% consume the recommended five or more servings of fruits and vegetables;

- Only one third of the population consumes foods from all the food groups on a typical day, with less than 3% consuming foods from all food groups in at least the recommended amount;

- Many diets contain half the recommended amount of magnesium and folic acid. As many as 80% of women who exercise may be iron deficient and the average calcium intake is two thirds of the RDA and

- The average calcium intake of teenage girls resembles that necessary for 3-5 year olds.

With today's hectic schedules, you are lucky to grab three meals a day, much less all the servings of fruits and vegetables that health guidelines recommend. But to fight everything from heart disease to breast cancer to obesity, experts agree that you should eat at least five daily servings of fruits and vegetables, nine being ideal, and in a variety of colours, which reflect different protective nutrients. One serving equals a piece of medium-size fruit; a half cup of fresh, canned, cooked or frozen fruit or vegetables; a quarter cup of dried fruit; or a cup of raw, leafy vegetables.

Believe in how much you need to eat

At breakfast time

What you must not do is spike your insulin in the morning with sugary cereal, a bagel or a Danish pastry, because you will be tired and hungry later in the day. Instead, opt for a breakfast that is rich in protein and complex carbohydrates. For example: eggs (not fried) on whole wheat toast. A high fibre, low sugar breakfast is especially crucial because it gradually raises your insulin level, leaving you in good shape for the rest of the day. A recent study compared groups of people who ate egg breakfasts versus groups of people that ate cereal or bagel based breakfasts. The results of the study showed that the egg eaters lost or maintained a healthier bodyweight due to eating fewer calories during the remainder of the day because their appetite was more satisfied, while the cereal/bagel eaters actually gained weight and would have been more prone to wild blood sugar swings and food cravings. Breakfast (breaking the fast), is the most important meal of the day. Don't forget that you wouldn't have eaten for 6-8 hours, maybe more, so a healthy breakfast is essential for weight maintenance and mental energy.

At lunch time
Under eating especially at midday can backfire on you. For example, if you just have a salad at lunch, which includes just a plate of lettuce, this may make you feel full temporarily but you'll crave those calories later, guaranteed. Eating every 2-3 hours after breakfast will keep the metabolism high, just so long as you are eating sensibly. For example, your snacks should be fresh fruits or low fat yoghurts, etc. The debate about eating late at night should never be an issue either, so long as the foods are healthy and the quantity is in moderation, but people tend to snack and binge on junk foods. It's fine to include salads with your meal, but save main-course salads for dinner. As for portion control, especially with a whole foods diet (i.e. with vegetables, whole grains and healthy protein), you have the freedom to eat until you're full. On the other hand, flour based products, like pasta and bread or refined foods like white rice, require more attention because these foods affect your blood sugar so keep the portions small (i.e. half a bagel, a cup of whole wheat pasta, etc.). Why not toss tuna and avocado with olive oil and lemon juice and pile it on a slice of whole grain bread?

For an evening meal
Adding protein, like chicken or fish, with plenty of green leafed vegetables will suffice. Overeating, on the other hand, is what got us here in the first place so moderation is key and making more sensible choices is paramount. If you can justify a 'not so good choice' by saying that you will work harder with the exercise then that is your choice, justification being the operative word.

Snacks in between
Eat plenty of fresh fruits or low fat yoghurts, etc.

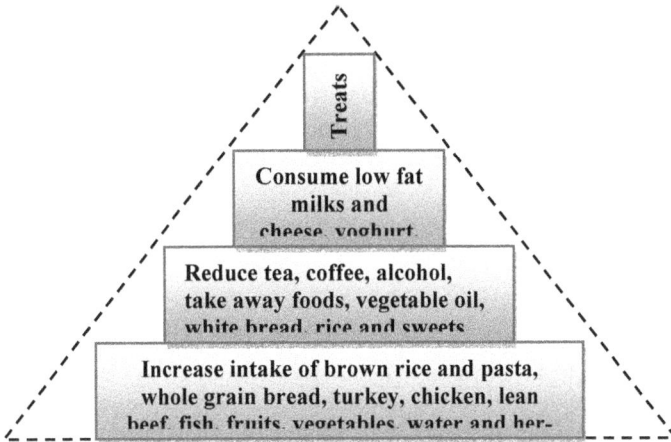

Lifestyle Challenge food pyramid

60

How should you eat?

As you enjoy the new found energy your new food choices gives you, try and remember that, when it comes to controlling emotions, how you eat is just as important as what you eat. When we look at the whole picture of food, with stress and mood, we need to include a lot more than just avoiding junk food.

Jack Challem, personal nutrition coach and author of The food-mood solution, agrees. "Part of this process comes down to two words - be mindful," he said. "People forget this all the time, especially when they're swept up by stress."

So, as an example, for your next meal, don't rush your meal in front of the computer. Sit down and savour the tastes with each mouthful and eat more slowly. It takes 20 minutes for the brain to sense fullness, so fast eaters tend to eat more than necessary and, in doing so they quite often wind up with an uncomfortably full belly.

Also, take time to pay attention to why you are eating. You could truly be hungry but make sure it's not just because you are lonely, bored or stressed. Therefore, if you make it a ritual to eat mindfully then you will have a new tool for staying calm and balanced. The key lies in the specific combinations and patterns of the foods you eat. By eating one food before another or with another, you can increase your calorie burn rate by 113% and that's how you can eat 3,500 calories and burn 4,000 or more. Put simply, by eating mostly what you're eating now but re-arranging your food into different combinations and patterns, you'll reach your ideal weight safely in record time. Just by altering and re-arranging your food combinations and patterns, you achieve 24/7 calorie burn to effortlessly and safely melt away excess fat.

Food enzymes begin the process of digestion in your stomach. If there are no food enzymes, your body must produce additional digestive enzymes, which results in fewer metabolic enzymes. If you eat a diet containing at least 70% of raw foods, you're providing these vital enzymes. Congratulations! Cooking or processing food above 118 degrees Fahrenheit destroys all food enzymes.

If your diet consists mainly of cooked or processed foods, your body's storage of metabolic enzymes will be converted into digestive enzymes. The lack of food enzymes puts a heavier burden on the body to generate adequate enzymes to complete digestion. Eating every 2-3 hours after breakfast will keep the metabolism high, just so long as you are eating sensibly i.e. your snacks are healthy options. For people with weak digestion, it is best to make food combinations as simple as possible. The more you can adhere to a simple mono-diet (i.e. eat one type of food at any one meal), the better your digestive system will cooperate.

What nutrients your body needs
Hone in on nutrients most known to boost stress coping ability and try to incorporate more foods containing B vitamins, folate, omega-3 fatty acids and magnesium into your diet. Deficiencies in these nutrients are linked to depression which will, inevitably, lead to more stress. Magnesium, for instance, helps muscles relax, helps you fall

asleep and stimulates production of GABA, a neurotransmitter that eases anxiety and nervousness. Stress also prompts your body to excrete more Vitamin C, which is why this vitamin is almost always required as a supplement. So go ahead and add a few extra berries to your morning oatmeal. Antioxidants should also be considered and if you remember me mentioning cortisol, which sets off chain reactions in the body that can damage brain cells and memory, adding these antioxidants will help fight that damage.

Good-mood foods
There's no such thing as a chill pill but certain foods contain body boosting nutrients that will help soothe stressed out nerves. Talk to your doctor about proper dosages if you only take supplements because, as always, it is possible to get too much of a good thing.

Stress soothers
Make the revamp of your daily food choices complete with an emphasis on whole foods (meaning unprocessed and unrefined) and eat them in frequent enough intervals to ward off fatigue and irritability. They'll help your body mellow existing stress and anxiety and set you on the right path for overall health.

Lifestyle Challenge recommendations, just for you

- Don't discount the role of liquids in your dietary audit because, if you are like the majority of people, you may turn to caffeine to jumpstart a sluggish day. What millions don't understand is that it can do more harm than good as it boosts the production of adrenaline, another stress hormone;

- Dependant on where you are during the day, in the house or at the office, it can get quite stuffy and it's easy to get dehydrated without noticing. If you always have a glass of water and sip it regularly you won't get the urge to be constantly making cups of tea and coffee, which will dehydrate you more and often lead to eating something alongside;

- Throw a cup of blueberries in your cereal every morning to get two servings right away or include two fruits or vegetables in every meal, like a salad with mandarin oranges, and then eat another as a snack. In this case, no matter what, you will get at least seven servings a day;

- With reference to vegetables, you can incorporate produce powder into yoghurt, soups and smoothies by adding a powdered vegetable supplement into your morning shake. All these added extras to make it easier are all available at health food stores around the world;

- Steaming vegetables makes them easier to digest and helps you absorb more nutrients, but just be careful not to overcook them. A good marker is that if the vegetables lose their vibrant colour, chances are they've also lost many of their vitamins and

- Your body has mechanisms for setting your weight where it wants it to be, which can best be described as similar to the way you set the temperature of your house with a thermostat. So the right tool for the job of losing weight is one that changes your body's set point, so you need to change your metabolism.

Re-energise the digestive system
Recommended for you is a 24-hour cleanse to re-energize the digestive system, which will sharpen your concentration and focus and improve your sleep patterns.
More importantly, it will allow nutrients to be better absorbed into your whole body, which will ultimately provide you with more energy.

1. Drink the juice of one lemon in fresh water during the morning hours;

2. 10-30 minutes later, consume any fruit or vegetable (juiced yourself) or fresh, raw vegetables in boiling water – soup;

3. Water (distilled) should be more than the recommended daily amount. Shoot for approximately ten glasses;

4. Throughout the 24 hours, you may consume any kinds of vegetables prepared as in number two, but the fruit should be one serving and just one kind, no combinations and

5. No salt is to be consumed throughout.

It will vary with each individual, but normally it should take between 1-3 days. You will know how it has gone if you are constantly on the toilet after each meal and if you are not then perhaps you should continue after the 24 hours, but definitely complete the cleanse once or twice a week. "Regardless of the time it takes for your initial cleanse to produce the desired results, going through this cleansing process will become easier and easier in subsequent weeks and your system will become cleaner and healthier as time goes on," says Christopher Guerriero, author of Maximize Your Metabolism.

Nutrition tips and diet information from different sources often conflict with each other, so you should always check with your doctor first.

Below is your next Lifestyle Challenge that you can begin immediately:

Lifestyle Challenge 5

1. I will attempt to cleanse my body of toxins prior to beginning this program;

2. I will eat a healthy breakfast to kick-start my metabolism;

3. I will eat the right foods at the right time and limit my processed foods;

4. I will eat more than 3 healthy meals per day in order to lose weight;

5. I will carry a bottle of water everywhere, drink hot water and lemon or un sweetened iced teas for their anti-aging antioxidants;

6. I will eat lots of fresh whole fruits and vegetables or make smoothies;

7. I will eat smaller servings of high fat/high calorie foods or just simply replace them with healthier foods or eat them less often;

8. I will pay attention, enjoy my food and eat more slowly, not in front of TV;

9. I will not eat fried food or take away meals and choose my meals at home or at the restaurant more wisely by eating more grilled food etc;

10. I will definitely eat more protein (chicken, turkey and fish) on a daily basis;

11. I will remember that alcohol has many hidden calories and

12. I will make my snacks healthier with tuna, chicken salad, etc.

Do not continue until you have written these down or cut them out to keep safe. You are now more than on your way to success. You are over half way there.

In the next chapter it will be revealed to you how certain movements, that are progressed gradually, will get you the results that you need.

A LIFETIME OF WEIGHT CONTROL

"You must have long range goals to keep you from being frustrated by short range failures."

- Charles Noble

Make today's society yesterday's news

If you believe that calorie restriction alone can help you achieve all that you desire for long lasting results, then let me put out your fire. This belief alone is a short sighted and incomplete approach to a complex problem. What is required is a complete change in lifestyle habits to achieve better health, better body composition and results that last.

Before this subject is addressed fully, you must ask yourself the following questions:

1. How active was I when I was younger?

2. What activities have I tried in the past?

3. What did I enjoy doing the most? and

4. How active am I now and how can I step it up a gear?

Once you have answered those questions, then you will have some idea of why I say that you must move to get to where you want to get to. But, before we do that, maybe we should take a look at how society has changed over the years and, more importantly, how we have let society rule us. We must acknowledge that at present, the majority of us own a car and people never used to go anywhere before without walking, cycling or running to wherever they wanted to go. At work and at home we have computers where we can tend to spend many minutes or hours just sitting there. We text, phone and generally communicate with friends and family that possibly live just around the corner or within walking or cycling distance.

At schools and with children is where the education needs to start. Instead of them sitting in front of the TV or Play Station for hours on end exercising their wrists or backsides, they should be playing all sorts of games and sports close by the house with their friends. They should be climbing trees (safely), making play dens, tree houses or just simply playing hop scotch or skip in the back garden....where did all that go? There seems to be less value for physical education these days during school hours, let alone after school programs. So what chance do we have in moving our way to a healthier future with our families?

Different types and amounts of physical activity are required for different health outcomes, which will be explained in detail in this chapter. Take a look at the difference between activity and inactivity:

Physical activity is defined as any bodily movement produced by skeletal muscles that require energy expenditure. Michael Van Straten, author of Super Radiance Detox, suggests that "with weight bearing exercises, you can prevent osteoporosis, a life threatening and ageing disease." He also states that "one in three women and one in twelve men will develop osteoporosis and tragically, it's happening in younger and younger people."

Physical inactivity is of course a lack of physical activity but it is an independent risk factor for chronic diseases. It is estimated to cause approximately 1.9 million deaths globally.

Physical activity and health:

- Is a key determinant of energy expenditure and thus is fundamental to energy balance and weight control;

- Reduces the risk of coronary heart disease and stroke;

- Reduces risk of Type II diabetes and

- Reduces the risk of colon cancer and breast cancer among women.

Resting metabolic rate
Resting metabolic rate (RMR) is the number of calories it costs for you to keep your heart beating, your lungs breathing, your brain and liver functioning, and all your cells alive and well at complete rest. RMR accounts for approximately 65% of your total daily calorie needs.

Of the factors you can control, the main one that affects your RMR is the amount of lean body mass you have.

Lean body mass (which includes muscle tissue) is very metabolically active and accounts for 75-80% of your RMR. People who have more muscle on their bodies burn more calories than people who have more fat on their bodies because at rest, one pound of muscle burns up to 70 times more calories a day than a pound of fat. What can you do to keep your metabolism revved up?

By regular resistance training 2-3 times per week, older women and older men can recover 10-20 years of loss respectively, with just two months of resistance training three times per week. Resistance training may include any muscle toning exercises, but when it comes to ageing and muscle loss, if you don't use it, you will lose it.

In addition to building muscle, which is more metabolically active tissue, very intense exercise sessions can speed up your RMR for several hours after you stop working out. So, people who have more muscle AND are training very hard most days of the week need a lot more calories just to maintain their internal physiological functions at rest. Some of these easier workout strategies are explained in more detail later in this chapter.

Move forward with movement and avoid the health scares

Avoid sitting around and try to be the first one to leap up and help with whatever needs to be done. Sitting around not only leads to eating, but it also promotes an energy slump, which will lead to more sitting around. Try and fit in your usual trip to the gym or activities when you can or go out for a quick walk every day, especially after a meal. Your activity or excuse to move could be anything to get the blood pumping and get you out of your chair.

A study of more than 13,000 men and women over an eight year interval indicated that even modest amounts of exercise substantially reduce the risk of death from heart disease, cancer and other causes. Therefore, if we avoid movement, then the opposite effect will be produced and we cannot attempt to balance metabolic activity, which is extremely important with weight loss.

Main excuses about exercising
Only one in four Americans exercise regularly and their reasons for not exercising are: time, boredom and pain. Let's look at them individually and bare in mind that generally there is a solution to almost any given problem:

- **Time** - You have 24 hours in a day. You sleep, you can spend a lot of time working, but you can generally lounge around alot too;

- **Boredom** - Prevent boredom by trying activities that you are interested in and

- **Pain** - You should only progress your exercise at a comfortable rate for you and when your body feels that it has reached a plateau.

At all times you have to be honest with yourself and if you have tried certain methods before, whether it be a diet or a certain exercise or activity, then maybe you have to stop saying "I've tried EVERYTHING" and admit that those things were more than likely the wrong things.

Light a fire
When it comes to metabolism, the value of exercise goes beyond the amount of calories you burn. Resistance training builds muscle and regular, sustained movement supports your thyroid, lowers inflammation and improves the rate at which insulin can move blood sugar into your cells, so there's more available as fuel and less sugar circulating in the blood to be turned into fat.

Sweating
Toxins are accumulated through rapid weight loss and, when you burn fat, the toxins it stores enter the bloodstream so the solution is turned to sweat. Your body excretes toxins and waste in perspiration and if you don't sweat, it can only be compared to not going to the bathroom. Regular exercise should make you sweat. Losing weight gradually, without crash dieting, will also help prevent your bloodstream from becoming a toxic dump.

69

Prioritising

Prioritising exercise is essential for weight loss, but that doesn't mean you have to become a gym rat. You simply have to do what fits into your life, even things you can do at home, so long as you get your heart rate up. It is common knowledge to all personal trainers, life coaches and others that the biggest obstacle for anyone wanting to begin a new weight loss program is how to get started, whether it is too intimidating or they just don't know where to start. If you are already doing some form of exercise or activity and for some reason you feel that what you have chosen is becoming a chore rather than a pleasure, then you need to remember three important things:

1. You have to do the exercises and/or activity for long enough to feel the benefits;

2. Results will come if you work at them for long enough;

3. A calorie is a unit of heat and therefore you must increase the heat to burn the fat and

4. Try and find the right things for you.

Which time of day is best for you?

As we have established, your body needs to move and this movement needs to become a habit. It should be no different to other actions that have become a part of your life. People who exercise in the morning are 40% more consistent than those who exercise later in the day and the key to long term weight loss is to commit to something and stick with it for the long haul and become consistent. When you're busy or stressed out, exercise is often the first thing to go but you are more likely to stick to your plan if you treat it as a can't miss meeting. Try marking your workout on your calendar or set yourself a reminder. Of course the time of day you work out depends on your routine but routines can be changed, whether you get up earlier or eat later, you can change and that choice, just like whether you want to lose weight successfully or not, will always be yours. Positive thinking and positive doing is how success is achieved and without paying attention to both, you may continue to struggle. There must be positive thinking and positive action. It is important at this stage to remind you of the major advantages to any exercise and how it can significantly reduce the risks of:

*   Stroke;

*   Diabetes;

*   Osteoporosis;

*   High blood pressure and

*   Stress and depression.

There are also several psychological benefits, including feeling better, sleeping better and an increased outlook on life in general. Many of the benefits and risks have been covered previously.

A calorie diet, with & without exercise...Revealed!

By now you should be realising how important exercise is but, to be honest, I have only just scratched the surface. Where is the evidence to suggest the effects of alternating calorie diet with and without exercise in the treatment of obesity? James Hill and colleagues from the Department of Paediatrics at Vanderbilt University in Nashville completed a study using moderately obese women who were randomly assigned to an alternating or constant calorie diet with or without aerobic exercise.

- Both of the diets provided an average of 1200 calories per day over a 12 week period;

- The women who exercised walked five days a week;
- All subjects participated in an intensive outpatient   behaviour modification program.

At the end of the study, exercised subjects had greater reductions in body weight and body fat percentage than the non-exercised subjects. Exercise was clearly beneficial in weight-loss therapy. This study involved the behaviour modification program which would have included changing the mindset about junk foods, drinking soda and eating in moderation.

Important: It's not how many calories you can burn per exercise, but how many calories you burn 24-7.

Eat & drink before, during & after exercise for more energy

- Before - If you're exercising for less than an hour, a bagel, toast, plain pasta, a banana or crackers are all good carbohydrate choices one to two hrs prior to exercise;

- During – Sports drinks, bananas or sports bars or just plain water are good options and

- After – One to two hours after exercising your priorities are carbohydrates and, of course, replenishing the fluids lost during your workout.

Research shows that it makes no difference in performance whether you drink your carbohydrates or eat them. Drink at least one glass of water before and after your workout and every 10 to 15 minutes during your workout to replace fluid lost in perspiration.

You will want higher intake of minerals (particularly electrolytes) and water soluble vitamins (vitamin C and all of the B vitamins) since you will be using them up and sweating them out at an accelerated rate.

As a side note, instead of drinking high sugar sports beverages you might want to consider just adding liquid trace minerals to your water.

Overleaf is an example of a training day diet - A 2400 calorie goal (Follow a similar diet 6 days/week; then have one relaxed day)

Meals	Prot (g)	Carbs (g)	Fat (g)	Cals (g)	Fibre (g)
Breakfast					
Egg sandwich (1 egg, 1 slice of medium sized chicken sausage, one slice cheese on whole grain bread)	24	30	14	330	4
1 kiwi	1	12	0	46	2
Water or unsweetened green tea					
Mid morning meal					
½ cup fat free ricotta cheese mixed with 1 cup vanilla yoghurt, ½ cup frozen fruit of choice (thawed) and ¼ cup chopped walnuts	30	48	20	474	6
Water					
Early afternoon meal					
Whole wheat sandwich (1/5 Ib lean meat: turkey breast, roast beef, lean ham, chicken breast or tuna, lettuce, spinach, slice cheese)	28	35	12	339	7
1 piece fruit (grapefruit, kiwi, mango etc.)	1	23	0	84	4
Water					
Late afternoon meal					
¼ cup chopped pecans, ¼ cup raisins, 1 hard boiled egg	12	32	24	377	5
Late Day Training Session					
Post training recovery meal					
Post workout recovery shake with 1 frozen banana, 2 tbsp pure maple syrup, 20g whey protein powder, 1 cup skimmed milk	30	67	0.5	386.5	2
Dinner					
¼ Ib organic lean meat (eye round steak, chicken breast, pork tenderloin, fish etc	26	0	5	149	
1 small- medium ear of corn	3	26	2	122	4
Steamed vegetables (unlimited)	2	8	0	34	2
Spinach salad with olive oil dressing	1	8	10	120	2
Water					
Totals for day	158	289	87.5	2461.5	38

Macronutrient profile (Fibre excluded from calorie count)

Prot = Protein 25.7%
Carbs = Carbohydrates 42.3%
Fat 32.0%

Exercise your mind & body:

1. Exercise increases your metabolism;

2. Exercise creates a caloric deficit without triggering starvation mode;

3. Exercise helps you sleep better and manage stress better;

4. Exercise (strength training) tells your body to keep the muscle while dieting causes muscle loss;

5. Exercise increases bone density;

6. Exercise helps prevent diabetes, controls blood sugar and improves insulin sensitivity;

7. Exercise improves cardiovascular health;

8. Exercise improves mood, helps relieve depression and increases self esteem;

9. Exercise increases mobility and quality of life as you get older and

10. Exercise helps you keep the weight off long term.

Preventing injuries at all costs

Most injuries occur to ligaments, tendons and muscles, with only about 5% of sports injuries involving broken bones. Most frequent sports injuries are sprains (injuries to ligaments) and strains (injuries to muscles) caused when an abnormal stress is placed on tendons, joints, bones and muscle.

Ways to reduce injury:

- Wear the right gear - Wear comfortable sports clothing and appropriate footwear;

- Increase flexibility - Stretching exercises before and after exercise can increase flexibility;

- Strengthen muscles – Adding resistance exercises to your workouts strengthens the muscles;

- Use the proper technique- This should be reinforced during the initial stages;

- Take breaks – Certain rest periods can reduce injuries and prevent heat illness;

- Stop your workout - If there is pain and

- Avoid heat injury - By drinking plenty of fluids before, during and after exercise. Decrease or stop during high heat/humidity periods and prevent heat injury by wearing lighter clothing.

Post injury

The moment you realise you've injured yourself, you'll need to take some steps to secure a full recovery later on. One of the most effective methods of treatment is R.I.C.E.R.

- Rest – This will help to slow down the blood flow to that area of the body and prevent any further damage;

- Ice - The most common recommendation is to apply ice for 20 minutes every two hours for the first 48-72 hrs;

- Compression – Helps reduce bleeding and swelling around the injured area and provides support for the injury. A wide, firm, elastic compression bandage can be used;

- Elevation – Raise the injured area above the level of the heart at all possible times, which will further help to reduce the bleeding and swelling and

- Referral - If the injury is severe enough, it's important that you consult a professional physical therapist or qualified sports doctor for a more accurate diagnosis and they'll be able to tell you the full extent of injury. As always, contact your paediatrician if you have additional questions or concerns.

How your posture can be the making of you

To excel in any physical activity and reap maximum benefits you need to have a solid foundation built on perfect form. People definitely take posture for granted, pretty much like breathing; they rarely consider it when exercising. Bad posture and incorrect technique can cause imbalances in the muscles, which leads to injury.

You can tell so much from a person when you look at their posture, as it can affect a person's presence, stature, and more importantly, their confidence. Here's exactly what it entails:

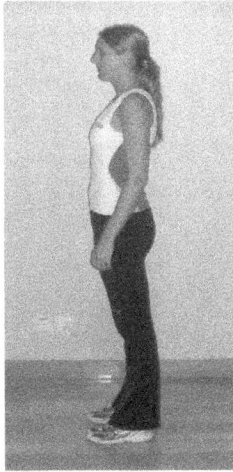

Head up, chest out, shoulders and arms relaxed.

Natural stance instructions:

1. Stand with your feet side by side, about shoulder width apart;

2. Raise up on the balls of your feet;

3. Now gradually lower your heels until they just barely touch the floor;

4. Push your sternum out slightly;

5. Tuck your chin in a little and

6. This is going to feel a little weird, lean forward ever so slightly from your hips.

HOW CAN YOU FIT EXERCISE INTO YOUR DAILY ROUTINE?

"Nobody who ever gave their best regretted it."

- George Halas

Breathe your way to health

As with posture, breathing during any form of exercise is often taken for granted, we obviously breathe all the time and often underestimate how much the way we breathe helps during our exercise routines.

Many people make the mistake of unconsciously holding their breath when doing a strenuous activity, but this in turn causes unwanted tension in the muscles, making the activity that much harder – whilst stretching is no exception!

Breathing properly promotes blood flow and increases the delivery of oxygen and nutrients to your muscles, which charges the whole body with more energy. Breathing is the most important physical principle to refine before an exercise or movement.

The following points should be considered;

- Relax the shoulders when breathing;

- Never hold your breathe and

- Breathe in through the nose for five seconds and out through the nose or mouth for five seconds.

Warm up, cool down & stretch

Your muscles, ligaments and tendons have to be warmed up so that they are less likely to be injured. You should try and pick a warm up activity or choose movements which call into action the muscles that you will be using during your workout.

The following should be included to ensure an effective and complete warm up:

Pre-exercise warm up
This phase of the warm up consists of 5 to 15 minutes of light physical activity and the aim is to elevate the heart and respiratory rate, increase blood flow and increase muscle temperature. If you are going to do an upper body workout, then start off at the top by gently moving your shoulders, then gently move your head from side to side and up and down. Then work your way down to the shoulders again with gentle arm circling, forwards and back and side to side.

Mobilise all the joints of the upper body in all ways until your muscles feel warm and your joints move more freely prior to the stretch phase.

If you are going for a walk or a run then you should be mobilising your lower body prior to the stretch. Move the hips, knees and ankles forwards and back and side to side to warm the muscles. Jogging forwards and back, side to side, raising the heels to your backside and knees to your chest are all different ways you can raise your heart rate and prepare yourself for the stretching phase.

Static stretching
The next 5 to 15 minutes of gentle static stretching should be used to gradually lengthen all the major muscle groups and associated tendons of the body, which increases your range of movement. This helps you move freely without restriction or injury occurring. The easiest way to remember how to breathe during a stretch is to exhale as you are moving into the stretch and inhale as you return to your original position. Breathing slowly and easily also helps to relax your muscles, which makes stretching easier and more beneficial. Check with a physician before doing any of the following: (Think about posture with ALL stretches. The head, shoulders and hips need to be aligned at all times).

Light stretches for walking, jogging, running and all lower body exercises:

1. Gluteus Maximus

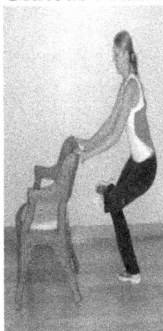

Buttocks and outer hip - Place the ankle just above the knee of the supporting leg, which should now be bent, and move your hips back and use support for balance if required.

2. Hamstrings

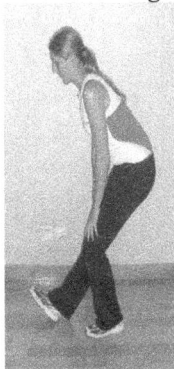

Back of the leg - Bend the back leg at the knee, lean forward with your upper body and feel the stretch more by raising the toe of the straight leg.

3. Quadriceps

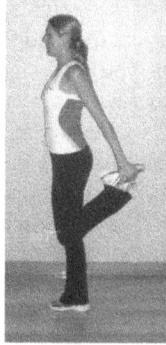

Front of the leg - Lift the heel of the bent leg towards your buttocks while keeping the thighs and knees close together.

4. Hip Flexors

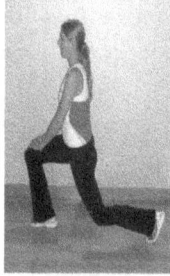

Front of the hip - Bend the front leg to approximately 90 degrees, the rear leg needs to be bent at the knee to feel the stretch at the front part of the thigh of the rear leg.

5. Calf

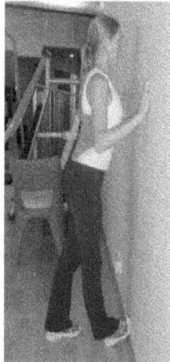

Back of the lower leg - Raise the toe of the front leg and use your body weight to increase the stretch of the calf of the straight leg.

Prior to starting your exercise program, you need to raise the heart rate even more. After the stretches have been completed, do all the movements that you did in the warm up phase but much quicker so that you can raise the heart rate and temperature of the muscles prior to the exercise program.

Post exercise cool down
The reasons why you stretch after exercise are very different to warming up, but very necessary for a number of reasons. Any strenuous activity, particularly weight lifting, causes a small amount of damage to the muscle and associated soft tissues. These small rips and tears are what force the muscles to grow when they begin the process of repairing themselves. Damaged tissue is replaced by stronger tissue, which, for up to 48 hours after exercising, often causes soreness. This is called DOMS or Delayed Onset Muscle Soreness. According to Brad Walker, a leading stretching and sports injury consultant with the stretching Institute "right after your workout your muscles are warm and elastic. The post workout stretching session affords you a second chance to increase your flexibility and range of motion, particularly around your joints. Regardless of the type of activity you should stretch all major muscle groups.

Walk away from your past & into your future

To get you started with movement, let us take a look at walking and just a few of its advantages. A walk may be just the thing you need to get you through your day. It can set the stage for inspired thinking and major mental breakthroughs because when you walk, you stimulate portions of the brain in the right and left hemispheres, giving you access to more areas of your brain than when you're sitting still. A million years of evolution have equipped our bodies to operate in an optimal way when we're walking and its part of our body's normal restorative process. Walking not only lowers your stress levels, it allows you to sleep better, improve your mood and of course it assists your diet in weight loss.

A few other advantages of walking are:

1. It is simple;

2. It is cost effective;

3. It is enjoyable;

4. You can walk anywhere;

5. You can walk at anytime;

6. It is low impact;

7. It is easy on your joints and

8. It is easy to fit into your day.

Technique for walking

Believe it or not, there is a technique for walking as there is for all activities of fitness and they all correlate to the correct posture.

Lift your head

A jutting head or chin can throw your neck and spine out of alignment, which in turn can cause strain. Therefore, you should lengthen the spine and the back of your neck to bring your shoulders to the proper position and allow your spine to unfurl. All of these pointers will help your body find its natural alignment.

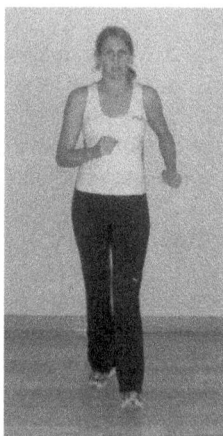

Engage your abdominals

A weak core, which puts excess pressure on the discs between your vertebrae, causes compression in the spine that can result in disc degeneration over time. Therefore, you should gently draw your navel in toward your spine to strengthen and stabilise your core muscles. All of these pointers will help tone abdominals, reduce pressure on your discs and will ultimately safeguard you against back injury. Better alignment of the pelvis, spine and rib cage protects your knees and lets your skeleton support your body more efficiently.

Don't squeeze

Overactive glutes work overtime even when they don't need to and this is often an unconscious attempt to stabilise the body. Clenched buttocks push the thigh bones forward, constricting the hips and lower back. Therefore, you should release the glutes as you walk and let your hips drift back slightly so they can sway naturally. All of these pointers will help reduce lower back strain and reduce tension. Plus, allow your abs to engage and stabilise the body rather than rely on your glutes to do the work.

Short stride

Over striding, which causes your leg muscles to work too hard, forces the knee into hyperextension, which can degrade the joint over time. Focus your energy forward and keep hips, knees and ankles in line by taking narrow, straight steps.

Progressive

Once the correct technique and posture have been mastered, then the pace and/or the distance can be gradually increased for more rapid results. Once the heart rate is increased then the body can become more conditioned. Working out too hard though, may boost inflammation levels rather than reduce them and, while some muscle soreness is warranted, if you're feeling exhausted or overly achy, rest a day before hitting the exercise again. All the walking in the world won't do you any good if you're tweaking your knee, jostling your spine or overtaxing your tight muscles.

While walking, the breathing should be deep, which will ensure that the lungs are being filled in a comfortable manner (during inhalation) and the exhalation should not be forced too much. The best advice is to breathe however you feel comfortable, although it is advised to try and breathe in through the nose and out through the mouth. Once you have been walking for some time and your body has become accustomed to it, then you can include a little jogging. For example, walk, jog and then walk again and it should be logged how far and for how long for each so that you can see your improvements along the way. I have provided you with some progressive programs to work from so that you can choose which one will be more suited to you personally.

Important: Even though it's great to have a workout partner, if you find yourself walking and having a nice conversation with your friend, then you can guarantee that you are probably not walking fast enough for the desired results.

Check with a physician before doing any of the following:

Light stretches for upper body exercises:

Triceps

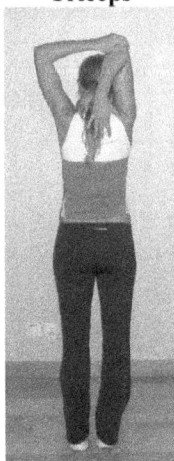

Rear View

Back of the arms
Bend the elbow of the arm that is over your head and push downwards on the elbow with the opposite arm.

Posterior deltoid

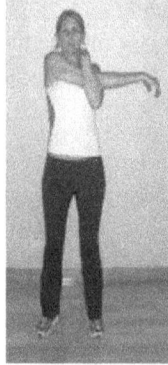

Back of shoulders
Pull the straight arm across the chest by grasping just above the elbow with the opposite arm.

Anterior deltoid & pectorals

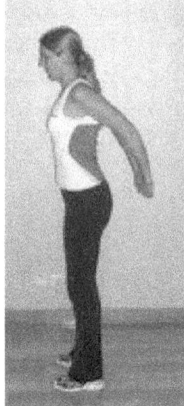

Front of the shoulders and chest
Expand your chest and pull your shoulders back while pulling your clasped hands away from your lower body.

The location has to be for your convenience

Outdoors

There are many advantages to walking outdoors compared to walking to a DVD or on a treadmill and the same principles apply for running too. Even though running places more stress on your joints, they can be limited greatly if you progress gradually from walking to running over a period of time chosen by you. Choose to walk somewhere soothing, like around a lake, instead of near a busy road and do your best to maintain an easy walking gait. Boost the intensity of your workout by using hills or by walking on grass, sand or trails. To quicken your pace, bend your arms to 90 degrees and swing them alongside your body and take quicker steps rather than long strides.

Treadmill

If you're starting out on the treadmill, then 10 to 15 minutes is enough to begin with and the recommended amount is around three times a week. The advantage of the indoor treadmill is that you can also work up to doing upper body exercises holding weights throughout the period of time you are on the treadmill and of course the advantage of using the incline button to work your leg muscles more.

In the home

If the gym scenario is not right for you and you don't really like the idea of people seeing you walking or running around your neighbourhood, there are certain alternatives. First of all, you could get someone to drop you off a set distance away and pick you up somewhere else. Remember, there is almost always a way around a particular problem or excuse. The choice of many people is to buy a fitness DVD. I remember a client who started this Lifestyle Challenge in the New Year who showed me a DVD that she had bought and tried it out and enjoyed it. The workout lasted for approximately 20 minutes. The best part about her motivation and realistic way of thinking was that she already knew that this wouldn't quite be enough but she knew that the DVD also came in 40 and 60 minute versions. You can get out of these DVD workouts what you need and in time your body and mind will tell you when you need to do more. You will either be very bored with doing them or you will get to a point where your results have reached a plateau and you will no longer feel you are progressing. My overall point is… at least you are moving and in some cases more than you were previously but you should continue to progress this over time with what exercise and/or activity you have chosen, until you reach your goal(s).

In the home workouts, you can use the DVD or a treadmill and you can also implement resistance exercises, which I will explain in more detail later in this chapter. In my opinion, the underlying factor is convenience to you yourself. Just as Douglas Brookes, author of *Your Personal Trainer* states "The opportunity to work out needs to be available at every turn in your daily schedule. It makes sense to be committed to exercise in a variety of ways that makes exercise easy, accessible and convenient. At every turn, the chance to agitate your body on a regular basis should be underfoot."

In the beginning, whether you are walking, jogging or running, you must keep your pace semi comfortable so that you can maintain it for a long period of time. I call this the active rest phase and you will understand this when I inform you of how low level interval training works. This method will give you a good platform and base to work from. When it comes to working in short bouts (low level intervals) at a later stage, your body will be aerobically accustomed and will adjust accordingly.

Warning:
The majority of people on new programs start off too fast too soon and therefore, can't physically or mentally continue and eventually they give up. You must remember that everything you change in your lifestyle must be maintained and everything you do **must be achievable** and progressed accordingly. Giving up in my opinion is not an option!

Why interval training will get you there quicker

Any form of exercise helps but there are ways you can rapidly increase your body's power to burn food calories, even when you're sleeping, by alternating periods of intense exercise with slower periods, which is known as interval training. This exercise pattern fine tunes your metabolism. You can choose to walk, jog, cycle, swim or row, it's up to you, and it basically consists of exercising for one minute at almost your maximum capacity and then for three minutes at moderate capacity (active rest). You can increase the time at maximum capacity and lower the recovery time (moderate capacity or active rest). Within the next Lifestyle Challenge I have developed workout programs that can be tried out when the time is right for you. If you attempt the programs and stick to them and progress accordingly, then this could be the difference between losing weight long term or sticking to a diet that will keep you bouncing right back to where you started. The programs I have developed for you are only examples but ultimately, when it comes to setting priorities for yourself, if you choose three intense workouts each week, it will be better than five gentler ones. It's as simple as that and, in actual fact, the more intense workouts will actually take up less time even though your warm up will need to be slightly longer to reduce the risk of injury. Don't toss the notion of long bouts of cardio out the window, but you should definitely consider adding short bursts of exercise into your day as a challenge. Maybe try for higher-intensity intervals once a week. For example, choose a landmark, such as the end of the block, and walk at top speed until you reach it. Repeat four to eight times on your walk.

Short versus long bouts
As with everything in the health and fitness industry, and of course the medical world, there are arguments for and against anything and everything. But with the debate about short, high intensity workouts versus long ones, the debate has been highlighted by John M Jakicic and colleagues from the *University Of Pittsburgh School Of Medicine* in Pennsylvania, USA. Their results suggested that short bouts of exercise may enhance exercise adherence and weight loss and produce similar changes in cardio-respiratory fitness when compared to long bouts of exercise.

Note: INTENSITY is about getting the most out of your cardio in the least amount of time, so revamp your cardio program with new energizing short burst intervals.

Building your strength will ensure long term weight loss

Did you know that you already possess the most powerful fat burner? It's your muscle. So why punish yourself and risk the loss of your fat burning potential? Adding just ten pounds of muscle to your body will burn off 62 pounds of fat over the next year, even while you are sleeping, and it will continue to do so day after day, week after week, month after month and year after year. Of course, cardiovascular exercise at 50% maximum heart rate for a minimum of an hour was always the preferred option for a personal trainer to tell his clients and, in some cases, that is true. What we all have to come to terms with now is: What gets better results and is quicker for weight loss?

In 2006, Stiegler, from sports medicine, suggested from his research that "strength training may have greater implications than initially proposed for decreasing body fat and sustaining fat free mass. Also, adding exercise programs to dietary restriction can promote more favourable changes in body composition than diet or physical activity on its own."

Strength training helps weight loss because of the following reasons:

- Strength training builds muscle;

- Strength training turns your body into a more effective calorie burner;

- Strength training helps prevent osteoporosis;

- Muscle burns fat and

- Muscle is more metabolically active than fat.

Just to reiterate what you read earlier, if you don't want to go to the gym and you want to avoid intimidating situations by doing certain things at home, keep a set of three and five pound weights in an accessible place at home for when you do your walking routine to a DVD or on your treadmill.

Resistant to resistance training
Toned simply means you have shed the fat that once covered your muscles and you can see your muscle definition, which gives your body a lean, tight shape. The only reason some women feel like they look bulky is because they have excess body fat while building muscle but they are simply not eating in a way that supports fat loss.

You won't bulk up

Facts:

- If you are female, you won't end up looking like a man;

- Women simply do not have enough testosterone to get big and bulky and

- You will achieve a lean, toned and firm body if you do regular resistance exercises.

Realisation

Now you can start to realise what your body has to offer you. Your body is the answer to the results you require, why do you think yoga has been around for so many years? This is because it works. Try practicing some strength training yoga moves, such as maintaining the plank pose, which is similar to holding yourself up during a full body push up. The plank pose not only makes your arms stronger, but it also works your back, abs, and legs at the same time and it is something you could do absolutely anywhere. This exercise, among others, is explained in more detail in a moment, but please don't get despondent. All of the recommended exercises that are within this book have an easier alternative way of performing the exercise and, of course, a harder version too.

Lean, toned, fit bodies have low body fat and a lot of lean muscle because strength training maintains and increases your muscle mass and decreases your percentage of body fat.

Targeting certain areas

Most of us have someone we admire or look up to but don't think for one moment that a celebrities toned arms or fabulous abs are created by some "magic" exercise that mysteriously melts fat off a particular area of the body or that they are any more happier with their bodies than anyone else. Now is the time to banish that myth once and for all.

1. There is simply no exercise that acts like a magic eraser to rid your body parts of unsightly fat, as that is not how the body works.

2. If you want to lose fat, you need to challenge all of the muscles in your body to boost your metabolism so that you lose fat all over.

Time saver

When it comes to fat loss, isolated, shaping exercises are generally a waste of your time and just because you feel the burn does not mean that you are burning the fat. One of the most effective ways in which to maximize your fat burning potential is through full body, short burst resistance training.

By working several muscle groups at once, short burst resistance training has the following advantages:

- Saves time;

- Skyrockets your energy levels and

- Incinerates fat and calories.

Strength or aerobic training?

I hope you realise by now that you cannot achieve permanent weight loss with just dieting alone. So, your choices are as follows:

- Diet plus strength training;

- Diet plus aerobic training and

- Diet, strength and aerobic training - advised for more rapid results.

Your level of intensity during your workout will dictate which one will work for you but the method will have to be convenient to your daily life. You should now be in more agreement that exercise should be an extremely important part of your life and in some respects it is a must if you want rapid results.

The right mix
The Lifestyle Challenges and progressive exercise programs will ensure that your routine is well-rounded, incorporating interval training (workouts of varying intensities) into your exercise routine for at least three times weekly and doing a minimum of 20 minutes of strength training (using your own body weight) two or three days a week. The intensity level will ultimately depend on where you are at now and what you will be comfortable with. Being realistic is the key to choosing where you start, we can only give you the choices, but please remember one thing - if you push yourself too fast, too soon, you will get despondent and you will more than likely give up, which is not an option!

In the next chapter it will be revealed to you how certain lifestyle changes can and will get you quicker results.

LIFESTYLE CHALLENGE WORKOUTS TO GET RAPID RESULTS

"Failing to plan means planning to fail. What are your goals?"

- Brian Tracy

MOVEMENT PLAN A:

Talk to your family doctor before you begin any type of exercise program. Your doctor can help you determine what kind of exercise program will be right for you.

- Walk outdoors;

- Walk on the treadmill and/or

- In your home to a walking keep fit DVD.

All of the above choices should be for a minimum of 20 minutes, at least three times a week or more. If your mind and body allows you to, you can incorporate some jogging with your walking routine for faster results, although this is your choice depending on your fitness level. If you choose to walk only, by the end of the 21 days (non-stop) you should be able to walk for 60 minutes non stop.

Whether you choose to just walk or walk and jog, you should build up to incorporate different ratios. For example, "1 in 3" is equal to one minute faster walking or jogging and three minutes of active rest walking. Of course "1 in 3" can also mean 20 seconds of short burst work to 60 seconds of active rest walking or even two minutes to six minutes, I'm sure you get the point. As your heart gets accustomed to what you are doing, challenge yourself further by changing the ratio yet again to "1 in 2" or "1 in 1," which basically limits your active rest time and you can ultimately keep increasing your short burst as much as you can sustain it.

Important notes: Whenever you active rest walk, you must walk with purpose as if you are late for an appointment. I have termed it as active rest walking because it must be a speed that you can maintain for a long period of time. Never forget the warm up and cool down phases that involve stretching.

MOVEMENT PLAN B:

Talk to your family doctor before you begin any type of exercise program. Your doctor can help you determine what kind of exercise program is right for you.

- In a gymnasium and/or

- In your home.

The most important aspect of this plan is good form. For example, you want to engage your abdominals and use them as much as you can, also breathe correctly and maintain good posture throughout the duration. It's better to do good repetitions and hold a good strict body position than to rush something, each time you try the exercises you will improve over a period of time, not forgetting the warm up and cool down phases that involve stretching.

Resistance: As you are already aware, by working several muscle groups at once, short burst resistance training:

- Saves time;

- Skyrockets your energy levels and

- Incinerates fat and calories.

Below is a table that briefly outlines the exercises to follow.

Groups	Exercises	Time	Remarks
Ex 1a - c	Plank	Maximum hold in 2 minutes	Keep the back straight at all times
Ex 2a - c	Sit-Ups	Maximum in 2 minutes	Keep the knees bent at all times
Ex 3a - c	Leg Squat	Maximum in 2 minutes	Make sure the knees don't go over the toes
Ex 4a - c	Push-Ups	Maximum in 2 minutes	Ensure the hands are in line with shoulders
Ex 5a - c	Stair Step-Ups	Maximum in 2 minutes	Stand up with a straight leg every time

You should attempt to do 2 minutes work on each exercise, even if you have to stop and carry on. Exercise 1a will be easier than 1b and so on. Your aim should be to hold good form and maintain good posture.

Exercise 1: Plank pose progressions

Exercise 1a

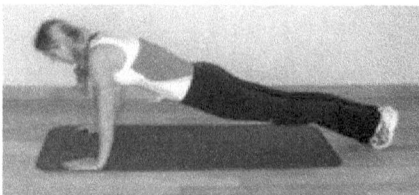

Hold your bodyweight up by your hands and feet.

Exercise 1b

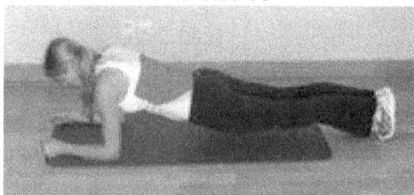

Hold your bodyweight by resting your forearms on the floor.

Exercise 1c

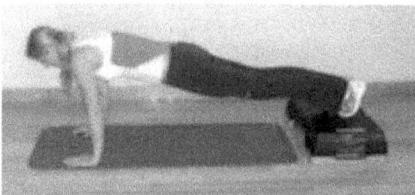

Elevate your feet on a platform to make it more difficult. Try the exercise on your forearms for more of a challenge.

Start - Start in an outstretched position as in all of the pictures.

- Your hands or elbows should be directly underneath your shoulders;

- Your feet should be together;

- Keep your back as flat as possible;

- Your head and neck should be in line with your spine and you should be looking at the ground slightly in front of you and

- Relax the tension from your shoulders.

Aim – To stay in this position as long as possible, just count those seconds and log down your achievements in your workout diary!

Tips & techniques - Remember to breathe, pull your belly button into your spine for maximum body tension and try not to let your hips drop or your buttocks to be raised too high.

Exercise 2: Sit-up progressions

All exercises start off by lying on your back with your knees bent and your feet flat on the floor.

Exercise 2a

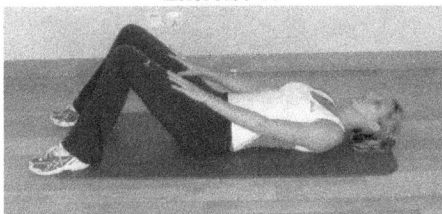

Exercise 2a

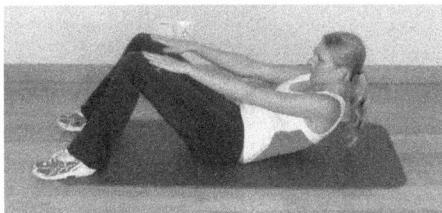

Exercise 2a - Touch the knees with the hands, hold for 2-3 seconds and return to the start.

Exercise 2b

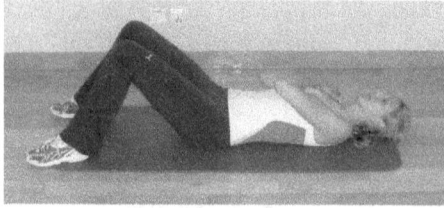

Exercise 2b

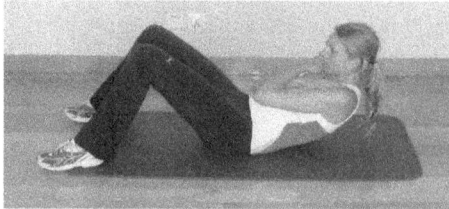

Exercise 2b – Keeping the elbows close in to the chest and lower back on the floor, curl up so that only your shoulders and upper back come off the ground. Hold again for 2-3 seconds and return to the start.

Exercise 2c

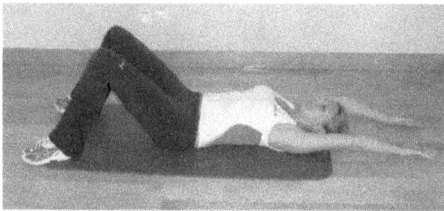

Exercise 2c

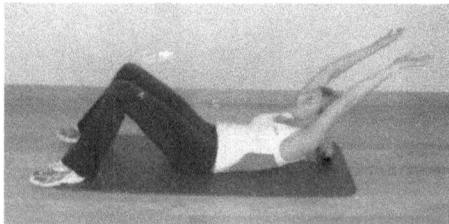

Exercise 2c - Extend your arms overhead, slowly raise your arms, head, shoulders, and upper back about 30 degrees off the floor. Hold before slowly lowering. Keep your arms straight, by your ears and in line with your head. Do not throw them forwards to help you. Add a weight in the hands if you can.

Note: To maximize ALL exercises, especially the abdominal ones, you can maximize the abdominal pressure by pulling in the stomach as if you are zipping up the fly on an extra tight pair of jeans. If you hold your stomach in while breathing out, keep sucking in the stomach more and more as you are breathing out.

You will feel your abdominals and lower back muscles contracting together and, in time, this will improve the support for your spine and lower back. This technique can be done anywhere, even while standing in a queue or sitting in your car. It should especially be utilised during exercise to accompany your body's postural alignment.

Exercise 3: Leg squat

Exercise 3a

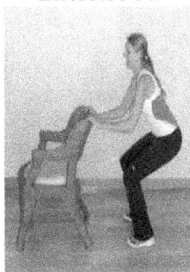

Exercise 3b

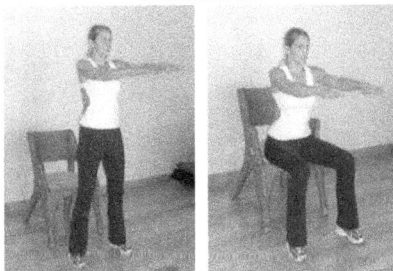

Exercise 3c

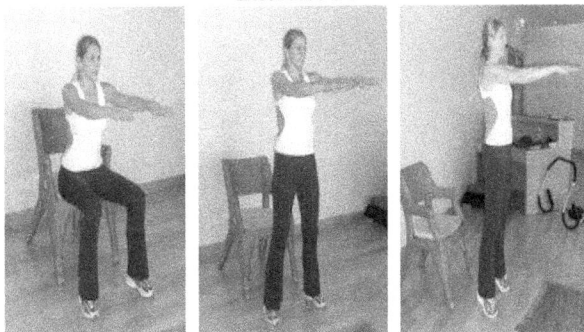

All of these exercises will tone the muscles in the back and front of your thighs and buttocks.

- You should stand with your arms fully extended in front of you for balance with your feet shoulder-width apart and your toes slightly pointing outwards;

- Keep your back straight and squat down until the tops of your thighs are almost parallel to the floor at 90-degrees. Be sure to keep your weight firmly over your heels and

- Rise back to the standing position, making sure that most of your bodyweight is through your heels. The chair should only be used as a guide.

Exercise 3c involves a heel raise at the end of the squat and can be done without a chair as long as you squat down to a 90-degree angle.

Note: As with any exercise, you can progress it accordingly, the balance aspect of it can be progressed by placing your arms across your chest and even closing your eyes, but remember to be safe. You can also add weights to your program by way of dumbbells or a barbell to increase your strength.

Make sure that your knees stay level or behind the toes at all times during the squat

Exercise 4: Push-Up Progressions

Exercise 4a

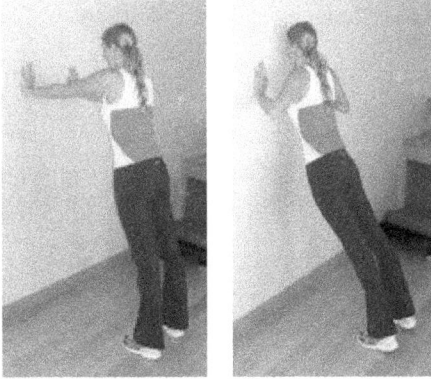

- Ensure the hands are in line with the shoulders and there is a straight line from your head, shoulders, hips and knees and tense the abdominals;

- Lower your body slowly towards the wall;

- Bend your arms and keep your palms in a fixed position;

- Your upper chest should be close to your hands;

- Straighten your arms as you push your body away from the wall and

- Relax the tension from your shoulders.

Try not to bend or arch your upper or lower back as you push up

Exercise 4b

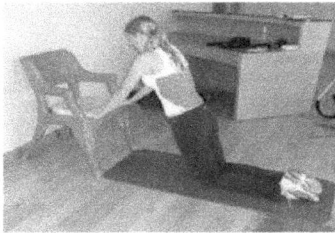

Utilise anything that is elevated off the floor, like a chair against a wall, your bed, your sofa or even your kitchen table, so long as it is secure. You will be testing your body strength more the closer it is to the ground.

- Ensure the hands are in line with the shoulders and there is a straight line from your head, shoulders, hips and knees;

- Keep the knees resting on the floor and keep your body straight;

- Lower your body slowly towards the elevated object;

- Relax the tension from your shoulders;

- Bend your arms and keep your palms in a fixed position and

- Then straighten your arms as you push your body up off the object.

Try not to bend or arch your upper or lower back as you push up

Exercise 4c

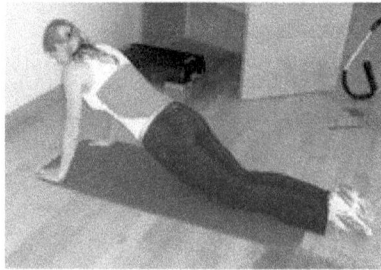

The push-up exercise has been gradually progressed against gravity and now you will be using the floor but still resting the knees. Try it without resting them if you can.

- Ensure the hands are in line with the shoulders and there is a straight line from your head, shoulders, hips and knees;

- Relax the tension from your shoulders;

- Keep the knees resting on the floor and keep your body straight;

- Lower your body slowly towards the floor;

- Bend your arms and keep your palms in a fixed position and

- Then straighten your arms as you push your body up off the floor.

Try not to bend or arch your upper or lower back as you push up

Exercise 5: Step-Ups

You can find stairs almost anywhere so make sure you do these exercises. In some ways step ups can be better for you than normal walking to get results quicker.

Exercise 5a

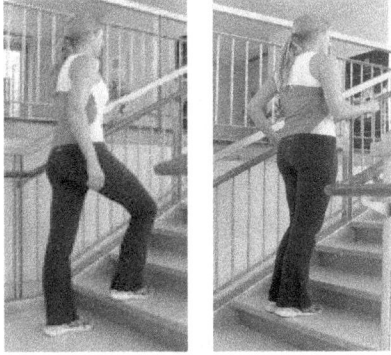

Exercise 5a is a simple step up and step down, changing the legs accordingly. Make sure you step up and straighten the leg fully.

Exercise 5b

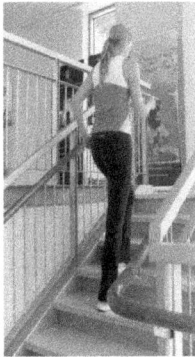

Exercise 5b is a simple walk up the stairs. Turn around at the top and return to the bottom, remembering to straighten the legs fully on each step.

Exercise 5c

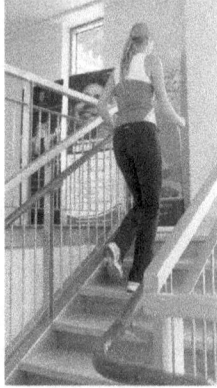

Exercise 5c is a simple jog up the stairs or you can alternate the jog with a walk up the stairs. Try and return to the bottom by walking backwards but remember to be extra safe. You are working your balance and muscles a lot more while walking backwards. Of course instead of walking backwards you can quite simply jog up and down for safety purposes.

Option 1: Complete Beginner, Diet & Exercise Combined

Walking only program for 21 days -

A daily/weekly walking log should always be kept for motivation and to ensure that you stick to your goals for the new you. Overleaf is an example of a walking only workout program for 21 days that will get yourself focused on your new daily routine, whether it is outside or on a treadmill.

If you choose to walk to a DVD for 20 minutes, try and do it once a day at the start of the program, twice a day in the middle and then attempt three times a day nearer the end.

This of course depends on the DVD and whether it includes resistance exercises or whether or not the time of the workout is longer than 20 minutes.

It's a good idea to get a bunch of DVD's that progress from 20 minutes to 40 minutes and then to an hour.

Day	Date	Distance	Time	Remarks on the walking only program
1	Jan 1	To local shops	**20 minutes**	Today I had to really focus on my posture
2	Jan 2			
3	Jan 3	On treadmill	**20 minutes**	Today I had to really focus on my technique
4	Jan 4			
5	Jan 5	DVD	**20 minutes**	My stretches are now becoming easier
6	Jan 6			
7	Jan 7	Around park	**30 minutes**	Started to walk with more determination today
8	Jan 8			
9	Jan 9	On treadmill	**30 minutes**	Felt good walking today
10	Jan 10			
11	Jan 11	Around park	**30 minutes**	My flexibility is improving
12	Jan 12			
13	Jan 13	20 mins out & back	**40 minutes**	Today I emphasized swinging my arms across my chest
14	Jan 14			
15	Jan 15	DVD	**40 minutes**	20 mins in the morning then in the evening
16	Jan 16			
17	Jan 17	25 mins out & back	**50 minutes**	My posture and technique are now perfect
18	Jan 18			
19	Jan 19	On treadmill	**50 minutes**	I feel so much more supple
20	Jan 20			
21	Jan 21	30 mins out & back	**60 minutes**	Felt good for achieving my goal

I realise that it states a set time out and the same time back on days 13, 17 & 21. Although this is an example, you should endeavour to walk back at a faster pace because you would inevitably be warmer and more motivated on the return phase. Walking every other day will give you ample recovery time and you should look forward to the rest time. Ultimately, you will be more than ready for the next workout day. If your day dictates that you cannot work out on a particular day, you can on two consecutive days.

104

Remember: This is Lifestyle Challenge 6 if you are a complete beginner to exercise. The previous other five challenges should already have been implemented into your mindset now and you should be well on your way to changing your life for the better. Out with the old and in with the new.

Option 2: A Beginner to Diet, Aerobic & Strength Work Combined

Diet, aerobic & strength program for 21 days –

A daily, weekly aerobic and strength log should always be kept to motivate yourself and ensure that you stick to your goals for the new you.

Overleaf is an example of a walking, jogging and strength program for 21 days, to get yourself focused on your new daily routine.

The aerobic work can be done outside or on a treadmill but again, if you choose to walk to a DVD, try to increase the intensity accordingly to encompass the program.

Day	Date	Workout	Time	Remarks on aerobic & strength work combined
1	Jan 1	Walk	**30 minutes**	Felt good just walking today
2	Jan 2	Strength	**20 minutes**	Today I concentrated on technique for exercises 1a, 2a, 3a, 4a & 5a
3	Jan 3	**Rest**		
4	Jan 4	Walk	**45 minutes**	Today I walked very fast for 1min and 3 mins briskly
5	Jan 5	Strength	**20 minutes**	I can now do more repetitions of exercises 1a, 2a, 3a, 4a & 5a
6	Jan 6	**Rest**		
7	Jan 7	Walk	**40 minutes**	Today I walked very fast for 1min and 2 mins briskly
8	Jan 8	Strength	**20 minutes**	I concentrated on technique for exercises 1a, 2a, 3a, 4a & 5a
9	Jan 9	**Rest**		
10	Jan 10	Walk	**30 minutes**	Today I walked very fast for 1min and 1 min briskly
11	Jan 11	Strength	**20 minutes**	I can now do more repetitions of exercises 1a, 2a, 3a, 4a & 5a
12	Jan 12	**Rest**		
13	Jan 13	Walk & Jog	**45 minutes**	Today I jogged for 1min and walked 3 mins briskly
14	Jan 14	Strength	**20 minutes**	My posture/technique are now fine tuned for all exercises
15	Jan 15	**Rest**		
16	Jan 16	Walk & Jog	**40 minutes**	Today I jogged for 1min and walked 2 mins briskly
17	Jan 17	Strength	**20 minutes**	I feel so much more confident with strength training now
18	Jan 18	**Rest**		
19	Jan 19	Walk & Jog	**30 minutes**	Today I jogged for 1min and walked 1 min briskly
20	Jan 20	Strength	**20 minutes**	I can feel that my body is now one unit and I look fabulous
21	Jan 21	**Rest**		

Remember: This is Lifestyle Challenge 7 if you have tried exercise before or you just realise that the strength (fat burning) exercises will get you faster results. The other 5-6 challenges should already have been implemented into your mindset and you will be closer than before to changing your life for the better. Out with the negative thoughts and in with positive ones.

Option 3: Accustomed To Diet, Aerobic & Strength Work Together

A daily, weekly aerobic and strength log should always be kept to motivate and ensure that you stick to your goals for the new you. Overleaf is an example of a walking, jogging and strength program for 21 days to get yourself focused on your new daily routine.

The aerobic work can be done outside or on a treadmill but if you choose to walk to a DVD, try to increase the intensity accordingly to encompass the program.

Day	Date	Workout	Time	Remarks on aerobic & strength work combined
1	Jan 1	Walk & Jog	30 minutes	Today I jogged for 1min and walked 2 min briskly
2	Jan 2	Strength	30 minutes	Concentrate on exercises1b+c, 2b+c, 3b+c, 4b+c, 5b+5c
3	Jan 3	**Rest**		
4	Jan 4	Walk & Strength	50 minutes	30 mins fast walk & all exercis-es 1b-5b
5	Jan 5	Jog	30 minutes	30 mins continuous fast jog (include ratios)
6	Jan 6	Strength	30 minutes	Posture/technique are now fine tuned for all exercises 1c-5c
7	Jan 7	**Rest**		
8	Jan 8	Walk & Strength	50 minutes	30 mins fast walk & all exercis-es 1b, 2b, 3b, 4b & 5b
9	Jan 9	Jog	40 minutes	40 mins continuous fast jog (include ratios)
10	Jan 10	Strength	30 minutes	Posture/technique are now fine tuned for all exercises 1c-5c
11	Jan 11	Walk	45 minutes	45 mins continuous fast walk (include ratios)
12	Jan 12	**Rest**		
13	Jan 13	Jog & Strength	50 minutes	30 mins continuous fast jog & all exercises 1b – 5b
14	Jan 14	Walk	60 minutes	45 mins continuous fast walk (include ratios)
15	Jan 15	Strength	30 minutes	My repetitions and sets are now high for all exercises 1c - 5c
16	Jan 16	Jog	30 minutes	30 mins continuous fast jog (include ratios)
17	Jan 17	Walk & Strength	60 minutes	30 mins fast walk & all exercis-es 1c – 5c
18	Jan 18	Jog	40 minutes	30 mins continuous fast jog (include ratios)
19	Jan 19	**Rest**		
20	Jan 20	Walk & Strength	60 minutes	30 minutes of each incorporat-ing all exercises 1b – 5b
21	Jan 21	Jog & Strength	60 minutes	30 minutes of each incorporat-ing all exercises 1c – 5c

If you think that walking is too easy for you and the rest periods are too often, then you can change them all around to fit in more jogging/running. But you should definitely try and rest in between strength sessions.

Try not to have two strength sessions on consecutive day. For example, there are two on days 20 & 21 but I have put that in because there is no strength for two days prior to that. As mentioned before, these are all examples of how you can implement walking, jogging and strength in a single program.

The allocated 20 minutes for strength can be increased and ultimately all timings can too. But this is why we have included the rest periods to make it more realistic because the rest time is very important so that your body can repair and grow accordingly and more importantly, so that your body can burn fat.

Your aim after the 21-day Lifestyle Challenge should be to implement a good hour a day to your exercise time and if possible, complete a good five days a week with two rest days in between, which will be dictated around your weekly plans. When it states, include ratios, this can be your choice i.e. you can choose 1 in 1, 1in 2, or 1 in 3 depending on how you feel on that particular day. The 20 minutes strength is pure work time and does not include the warm up, stretching or cool down but it's not bad to think that just by going through the exercise program twice you will be activating your fat burning muscles for only 20 minutes (actual work time).

Physiologically, you should complete the strength work prior to the aerobic work because large amounts of energy from the whole body can be expended while walking, jogging or running. Most of the body weight exercises are specific to local muscular endurance and will only use up energy from those specific target areas.

You should experiment and find out how you feel by doing aerobic first and then strength and vice-versa. It will ultimately depend on your intensity levels and how hard you work while walking, jogging or running and this will dictate how you feel when doing the strength work. Also, because some of the exercises I have chosen are specific to core strength, it is sometimes best to do these at the end of a workout. Fine tune to your specific needs by how you feel. These observations should all be recorded in your diary, which you will need to keep, so that you can look back at your performance and how you felt.

Remember: This is also Lifestyle Challenge 7 if you have tried exercise before or you just realise that the more difficult strength and fat burning exercises will get you faster results. The other 5-6 challenges should already have been implemented into your mindset now and you will be closer than before to changing your life for the better. Out with the negative thoughts and in with positive ones.

Lifestyle Challenges 6 & 7

I agree with the following:

- I will make time for exercising within my daily routine;

- I will definitely get up and move around more during the day;

- I will walk anywhere I possibly can, avoiding using lifts or escalators;

- I can begin to walk slowly and gradually progress to walking faster and further;

- I can walk anywhere, whether it is at home on a treadmill or to a DVD, or even outside;

- When I walk faster I will walk with conviction as if I am late for an interview;

- In time my body will know when I am ready to alternate walking and jogging;

- When I have tried ratio training and I reduce my recovery time I can jog further;

- I now know my own body can burn fat so I need to do the exercises in this book;

- I will attempt the exercises because they are easy to do and then progress in time and

- Even if exercising seems hard, it will become easier as I become more positive.

Only continue when you have written these down or cut them out to keep safe. You are now more than on your way to success, you're almost there.

In the next chapter it will be revealed to you how to:

1. Start your program;

2. Protect it and

3. Maintain it forever.

START YOUR PROGRAM, PROTECT AND MAINTAIN IT FOREVER

"Success is not the result of spontaneous combustion, you have got to set yourself on fire for it."

- Anonymous

Your past dreams are history

You must rise above everything that you thought to be correct before and eliminate all past beliefs from your mind before you can begin. You can certainly make gradual and small changes with your choices today in the here and now, which should only be positive. Your adaptation to today's society will help you become all that you deserve to be. Just remember that any change is better than nothing and that all choices you make from now on are yours and yours alone.

Take just one little habit that you know is not doing you any good and change that one thing. It could be something like eating a cookie every time you have a coffee or piling the food too high on your plate or simply not eating breakfast. It could be forgetting to prepare a healthy lunch to take to work so that you have to go out for a Subway mega-sandwich or fast food. It could simply be eating beyond your point of being satisfied at dinner time.

Whatever it is you choose, just focus on one little thing for now and build on that by changing your old habits for better ones. If you can, replace the majority of them over time and the sooner you can implement these strategies, the quicker you will get the results you deserve. Do the best you can but remember its progress not perfection. Give yourself the whole 21 days (non-stop) so that these thought processes and movement activities become a part of your daily, weekly, monthly and life long routine.

Remember 3 things:

1. Drastic weight loss means drastic life changes, which very rarely stick. That's why the weight piles back on afterwards. The 21-day Lifestyle Challenge is the only way to begin to achieve what you desire.

2. Successful weight loss is in those little changes you make one step at a time, one after the other, until they become part of your life. Use these 7 easy-to-follow steps wisely.

3. You can start the 21-day Lifestyle Challenge at anytime but you must be ready with no distractions and definitely no excuses. And remember that resolutions very rarely stick.

The truth of the matter is that no personal trainer, nutritionist, lifestyle consultant or mentor that you hold dear can possibly make any decisions for you now. The answer is already within you yourself.

Your new realisation and patience will get you there

A pound of fat is about 3,500 calories, so to lose one pound of fat in a week you have to eat 3,500 fewer calories in that week, which is only 500 fewer calories a day and not difficult at all. Or you have to burn off an extra 3,500 calories and we have already established that this is more than possible with all of the Lifestyle Challenges and their guidelines, by burning off calories by exercising or just by moving more.

Many experts believe you should not try to lose more than two pounds per week because losing more than two pounds in a week usually means that you are losing water weight and lean muscle mass instead of losing excess fat. If you do this, you will have less energy and you will most likely gain the weight back.

- **No brainer**
  The best way to lose weight and keep it off forever is to eat fewer calories and burn off calories with the exercises in this book. If you cut 250 calories from your diet each day and exercise enough to burn off 250 calories, that adds up to 500 fewer calories in one day. If you do this for seven days, you can lose one pound of fat in a week. It's easy math!

- **Influences**
  We are all responsible for how we influence others, especially our children. By setting values, morals and lifestyle patterns, our children will pass on to others what they have learned in their environment. Such choices greatly affect our future health patterns and those of our children.

- **Justification**
  You must always justify your actions and everything that you eat, drink, do or think. Once that is instilled in your head, which it should be by now, then you are a winner. You are a success and you are well on your way to becoming all that you have ever wanted to be and dreamed of.

Burning fat and transforming your body is simple, but you have to work at it. If you're willing to put the work in, you will take out the rewards but be patient because, as you know, all good things come to those who wait!

Combining it all as one

In this book we have been mainly focusing on weight loss itself, which is very important but what we tend to forget is that it is overall health that we should be focusing on. Even though contributing factors to death are all interlinked in some way, we should still look at the real causes of heart disease:

- Eating trans fats i.e. artificially hydrogenated oils;

- Cooking with heavily refined vegetable oils, such as soy, cottonseed, corn oil, etc. They are inflammatory inside the body and typically throw the omega-6/omega-3 balance out of whack;

- Eating too much refined sugar in the diet, including high fructose corn syrup;

- Eating too much refined carbohydrates, such as white bread and low fibre cereals;

- Smoking;

- Leading a stressful lifestyle;

- A lack of exercise and

- Other lifestyle factors.

Apart from smoking, heart disease and being overweight have the same contributing factors so if this means making small improvements to your meals and your habits, until they feel natural and a part of your new mode of thinking, then you'll surely reap the benefits forever.

When the time comes and your stomach is saying I need food, you have to give it something but it will be down to you what you give it. The secret to success for 'maintaining an optimum weight' is eating a little now when you first feel hungry rather than a lot more later when you're truly starving.

Snacking is the best way to maintain your blood sugar and weight. Some people think snacking is cheating or ruining your appetite, but all you are doing is eating in a measured way all the time. Healthy snacking keeps you from bingeing on a huge dinner after starving yourself all day. Why do you think it is that you see the skinny girl in the corner nearly always eating? The choices you make, as important as they are, will reflect on how you feel, how you function and if you know in your heart of hearts that those choices were better than before, then and only then are you on your way to winning.

Enjoy moving -

- Instead of heading to the fridge, put on one of your favourite songs, grab your training shoes, and do a few sets of all over body exercises;

- Need a change of scenery? Embrace yard work. Mowing the lawn with a push mower and digging in the garden will all get your muscles working. Do anything you can;

- Maintaining a regular yoga practice can enhance your weight loss regime, primarily by toning muscles and reducing stress. If this is your new choice of activity, aim to practice for at least one hour, two times a week and varying the type of yoga you do, from gentle to more intense styles;

- At this stage you shouldn't be thinking of any excuses, you should be on the road to being positive with the smart strategies that you have just revealed, strategies that you can ultimately start to adopt now;

- You should be thinking about boosting the intensity of your daily life with quality foods and safe exercises, complete with a good attitude and a realistic frame of mind and

- You should try and use your common sense at all times throughout the program. For example, walking up hills is better than on flat ground and swinging your arms across your chest will be better than not. Swimming is free and great on the joints.

Why not try something fun while getting in great shape at the same time? Maybe you could start hiking mountains or take up cross country skiing, snowshoeing or downhill skiing. The activity you choose is more than just fun and when the weather warms up, perhaps you could try out water sports like kayaking or canoeing or take up mountain biking.

Remember: Strength training has greater implications for decreasing body fat and sustaining fat free mass. Adding exercise programs to dietary restriction can promote more favourable changes in body composition than diet or physical activity on its own.

Road to success

- Eat healthily regularly;

- Cut out the JUNK carbohydrates and fats;

- Eat good old fashioned home cooking and avoid take away or ready meals that began in a science lab;

- Baking, boiling, steaming and stir-frying are examples of heart healthy cooking;

116

- Stop eating before you become stuffed, full and uncomfortable;

- Never go hungry, you'll find yourself nibbling on everything that comes your way so don't skip meals and

- Eat a piece of fruit on the way to the restaurant to put that appetite under control.

Remember that it's just the little things. As an example, the average American is gaining a minimum of 1 pound of weight each year and did you know that this is the result of eating just ten extra calories a day? So instead of depriving yourself of all your favourites, continue to enjoy them every once in a while. It's the little things that will make a difference. If you must have butter, have it on one slice not two. If you must have your caffeine, get used to black, decaf or organic coffee. Stop at the tenth chip not the whole bag, at least it will be justified.

Calories in, calories out –
To lose weight, you have to cut down on the number of calories you consume and start burning more calories each day. Calories are the amount of energy in the food you eat and some foods have more calories than others. But, foods high in fat and sugar are also typically high in calories. If you eat more calories than your body uses, the extra calories will be stored as excess body fat.

Making the transition from a bad fat diet to a good fat diet is easier than you would think. All you have to do is minimise your consumption of meat, full fat dairy products, fast food, and products made with partially hydrogenated oils, vegetable shortening, and common vegetable oils. Keep it realistic and achievable at this stage so that it doesn't become a chore but ultimately it becomes a natural part of your day. This first 21 days are the most important. All of the Lifestyle Challenges should be incorporated into your new daily routine to include:

1. Reasons why you want to lose weight;

2. Positive thinking;

3. Visualisation;

4. Goal setting;

5. New food choices;

6. Movement plan A and

7. Movement plan B.

Your present motivation level will dictate when to start your Lifestyle Challenges and incorporate them into your daily routine. It's pretty much down to you but the timing has to be right, if not perfect.

Michael Van Straten, author of Super Energy Detox explains that "you should just focus on putting one foot in front of the other and you'll be surprised at how quickly you become absorbed in what you're doing, and that will be the beginning of the regeneration of your energy."

If you think it will help, re-read this book, but you must adopt ALL of the strategies.

If you remember nothing else, remember this, something that I will never forget my grandfather saying to me: "No one person who has already achieved what they want in this life are any kind of superman or superwoman. They are not special in any way, shape or form. Of course they had motivation and the willpower to carry on, but we are all born with the same make-up." YOU have the same desire, just like my past clients, and now you have the same encouragement. I want you to be successful, in fact, I know you will be, but you yourself must believe, because if you believe in yourself then you will make it.

I wish you all that I wish for myself, and more!

info@wholebodyworkshop.com
www.wholebodyworkshop.com

REFERENCES

Section 1
Calle, E. E. "Body Mass Index and Mortality." New England Journal of Medicine (1999)

Willis, Judith. Drug Bulletin. Food & Drug Administration, 1996.

Packer, Lester, and Carol Colman. The Antioxidant Miracle. New York City: John Wiley & Sons, Inc., 1999. 185-196.

Section 2
Liao, K. Lih-Mei. "Cognitive-Behavioural Approaches and Weight Management: an Overview." The Journal of the Royal Society for the Promotion of Health 120 (2000): 27-30.

Packer, Lester and Carol Colman. The Antioxidant Miracle. New York City: John Wiley & Sons, Inc., 1999. 165-184.

Section 3
Van Straten, Michael. Super Energy Detox. Whitecap Books, 2003. 73.

Koh-Banerjee, Pauline, Mary Franz, Laura Sampson, Simin Liu, David R. Jacobs, Donna Spiegelman, Walter Willett, Eric Rimm. "Changes in Whole-Grain, Bran, and Cereal Fibre Consumption in Relation to 8-y Weight Gain Among Men" The American Journal of Clinical Nutrition 80 (2004): 1237-1245.

Segal-Isaacson, C.J. "First Major Study Examining Long-Term Followers of Low-Carbohydrate Diets." Division of Health, Behaviour and Nutrition. 2004.

Volek, J.S., M.J., Sharman, D.M. Love, N.G. Avery, A.L. Gómez, T.P. Scheet and W.J. Kraemer. "Body Composition and Hormonal Responses to a Carbohydrate-Restricted Diet." Metabolism 51 (2002): 864-870.

Ludwig, David, director. Optimal Weight for Life (OWL). Children's Hospital Boston. 10 Mar. 2008

Skov, A.R., S. Toubro, B. Ronn, L. Holm and A. Astrup. "Randomized Trial On Protein VS. Carbohydrate in Ad Libitum Fat Reduced Diet For The Treatment of Obesity." International Journal of Obesity 23 (1999): 528-536.

Saris, W.H., A. Astrup and A.M. Prentice. "Randomized Controlled Trial of Changes in Dietary Carbohydrate/Fat Ratio and Simple VS. Complex Carbohydrates on Body Weight and Blood Lipids: the CARMEN Study, the Carbohydrate Ratio Management in European National Diets. International Journal of Obesity 24 (2000): 1310-1318.

Astrup, A., G.K. Grunwald, E.L. Melanson, W.H.M. Saris and J.O. Hill. "The Role of Low-Fat Diets in Body Weight Control: A Meta-analysis of Ad Libitum Dietary Intervention Studies." International Journal of Obesity 24 (2000): 1545-1552.

Section 4
Ello-Martin, Julia A., Jenny H. Ledikwe and Barbara J. Rolls. "The Influence of Food Portion Size and Energy Density on Energy Intake: Implications for Weight Management." American Journal of Clinical Nutrition 82 (2005): 236S-241S.

Section 5
Johnston, Carol S. "Strategies for Healthy Weight Loss: From Vitamin C to the Glycemic Response." Journal of the American College of Nutrition 24 (2005) 158-165.

Anderson, James W., Tammy J. Hanna, Xuejun Peng and Richard J. Kryscio. "Whole Grain Foods and Heart Disease Risk." Journal of the American College of Nutrition 19 (2000) 291S-299S.

Thom, Susan. "Nutrition Facts to Help Consumers Eat Smart - Food Label Changes, Focus on Food Labeling" U.S. Food & Drug Administration. May 1993.

Schneeman, Barbara. "Whole Grains & Health" U.S Food & Drug Administration. 2005.

Garcia, OZ. The Balance. New York City: ReganBooks, 1998. 113-132.

Section 6
Nicola Reavley, author of The Encyclopedia of Vitamins, Minerals, Supplements & Herbs, how good is the average diet? 1998 13–17

Challem, Jack. The Food-Mood Solution: All-Natural Ways to Banish Anxiety, Depression, Anger, Stress, Overeating, and Alcohol and Drug Problems – And Feel Good Again. Hoboken, New Jersey: John Riley & Sons, Inc., 2007.

Christopher Guerriero, author of Maximize Your Metabolism www.MaximizeYourMetabolism.com, Unleash your metabolism, proper elimination begins with a thorough cleansing, 2005, 28-33

Section 7
Van Straten, Michael. Super Radiance Detox. Quadrille Publishing Ltd., 2002. 70-72.

Paffenbarger, R.S. "et al Reduced Risk of Death With Regular Exercise." The New England Journal of Medicine 314 (1986).

Hill, J.O., D.G. Schlundt, T. Sbrocco, T. Sharp, J. Pope-Cordle, B. Stetson, M. Kaler and C. Heim. "Evaluation of an Alternating-Calorie Diet With and Without Exercise in the Treatment of Obesity." The American Journal of Clinical Nutrition 50 (1989). 248-254.

Walker, Brad. <u>The Stretching Handbook</u> 3rd Edition (2007), 21.

Section 8
Jakicic, J.M. R.R. Wing, B.A. Butler and R.J. Robertson. "Prescribing Exercise in Multiple Short Bouts Versus One Continuous Bout: Effects on Adherence, Cardiorespiratory Fitness, and Weight Loss in Overweight Women." <u>International Journal of Obesity and Related Metabolic Disorders</u> 19 (1995), 893-901.

Stiegler, Petra and Adam Cunliffe. "The Role of Diet and Exercise for the Maintenance of Fat-Free Mass and Resting Metabolic Rate During Weight Loss." <u>Sports Medicine</u> 36 (2006), 239-262.

Road To Success
Van Straten, Michael. <u>Super Energy Detox</u> Quadrille Publishing Ltd., 2002. 54-58

INDEX

www.ingramcontent.com/pod-product-compliance
Lightning Source LLC
Chambersburg PA
CBHW022115280326
41933CB00007B/399